Racism in Europe

Racism in Europe

A challenge for youth policy and youth work

Edited by

Jan Laurens Hazekamp
Stichting Alexander, Amsterdam
and
Keith Popple
University of Plymouth

UCL
PRESS

First published in 1997 by UCL Press

UCL Press Limited
1 Gunpowder Square
London EC4A 3DE

and

1900 Frost Road, Suite 101
Bristol
Pennsylvania 19007-1598
USA

The name of University College London (UCL) is a registered
trade mark used by UCL Press with the consent of the owner.

British Library Cataloguing-in-Publication Data
A catalogue record for this book is available from the British Library.

Library of Congress Cataloging-in-Publication Data are available

ISBNs: 1-85728-257-4 HB
           1-85728-258-2 PB

Printed and bound in Great Britain by
T.J. International Ltd, Padstow, Cornwall

Contents

CONTENTS

CONTENTS

Acknowledgements

Producing a book that draws from contributors living and working in five different European countries and initially written in five different languages has demanded a great deal of organization, persistence and patience. We would therefore like to record our thanks to the contributors for their work and for producing it with expertise and enthusiasm. We would also like to thank our respective institutions and colleagues for supporting and assisting our endeavour.

Staff at UCL Press have provided constant help and encouragement and their tolerance during the book's production has been sorely tested.

Finally, we would like to thank our respective families and friends who have had much to put up with while we both wrote and liaised in the production of the book.

Notes on the contributors

Pablo Angel Meira Cartea is Professor of Environmental Education and Educational Intervention with Youth at the University of Santiago de Compostela (Galicia, Spain). His present research is in the environmental education of adults, social intervention with young people in rural environments, and youth policy and education in Galicia.

José Antonio Caride Gómez is Professor of Social Pedagogy and Director of the Department of Theory and History of Education at the University of Santiago de Compostela. He is engaged in research in education and rural society; education and cultural politics, education in Galicia, and education and "tiempos sociales".

Jan Laurens Hazekamp was until recently Senior Lecturer in Social Pedagogy at the Free University, Amsterdam. He has published extensively in the field of youth policy, youth culture and youth institutions. At present he is engaged in organizing youth research and consultancy programmes in which young people are directly involved. He is also Director of a governmental social work programme "Children at Risk in Russia". This collaborative project involves agencies in The Netherlands and the Russian Federation.

Lena Inowlocki is a sociologist at the University of Frankfurt am Main. Her areas of interest are qualitative–interpretative research and biography analysis. She is currently examining right-wing extremism and young people, and generational processes in migrant families.

Yvonne Leeman is a sociologist at the University of Amsterdam, lecturing and researching in the Faculty of Pedagogical and Educational Sciences. She previously worked in the Centre for Race and Ethnic Studies at the same university. Her main areas of interest are education, ethnicity and youth.

Rudolf Leiprecht is a lecturer and researcher at the University of Tübingen in Germany, and researcher at the Free University of Amsterdam. He has researched and published extensively in the areas of comparative studies of youth and racism, and intercultural education in The Netherlands and Germany. He is also a documentary film maker on themes connected with these studies.

Athanasios Marvakis is a psychologist at the University of Tübingen. He has conducted studies on youth and nationalism, youth exchanges, and young people and social inequality.

Jürgen Novak is Professor in Sociology at the Alice-Salomon-Fachhochschule für Sozialpädagogik und Sozialarbeit, Berlin. His main areas of interest are the sociology of social problems, social network analysis, and migration and Eastern Europe.

Keith Popple is Senior Lecturer in Community Work and Social Policy at the University of Plymouth, UK. Previously a youth worker and a community worker in multiracial areas, he has written widely on race and young people, and community work. He is presently engaged in researching the impact of theatre in health education in economically deprived communities, and in equal opportunity policies and practices in community work projects.

Gie Redig is Director of the Flemish Municipal Youth Services (VVJ). The Federation is a member organization for local govern-

NOTES ON THE CONTRIBUTORS

ments and undertakes surveys and training in all aspects of local youth policy.

Sawitri Saharso trained as a sociologist at the University of Amsterdam and was previously a lecturer at the Centre for Race and Ethnic Studies where her area of interest was ethnicity and youth. As a lecturer in the Department of Political Science and Public Administration in the Faculty of Social Cultural Sciences, she is currently engaged with various subjects including gender, ethnicity and the state.

Danny Wildemeersch is Professor of Social Pedagogy and Androgogy at the University of Nijmegen in The Netherlands. He is also engaged in teaching and research in the area of sociology at the University of Leuven in Belgium. His main focus of research is on adult and continuing education, and experiential learning and social change, including the situation of young people in The Netherlands and Belgium.

1

Racism, youth policy and youth work in Europe: a fragmented picture

Jan Laurens Hazekamp and Keith Popple

Introductory comments

In recent years a great deal of concern and interest has been shown by a wide range of individuals and organizations, as well as European governments, in the phenomenon of racism and young people. This concern has been demonstrated in a number of discussions at different levels that have attempted both to explain and to understand what has become one of the major social problems in Europe. However, less energy appears to have been devoted to counter racism, which has left its victims feeling as vulnerable as ever.

Our concern at this slow response arose during 1991 while attending the City Youth in Multi-Ethnic Europe Conference in Amsterdam, where we were able to debate with practitioners and policy makers from the European Union the role of youth policy and youth work in both encouraging and supporting cultural links and in combating racism. It was clear that although countries differed in their approaches there was much to be learnt from one another. At the same time we were aware that, while there was a substantial number of people expressing the need for progressive anti-racist action, there was a long way to travel to really begin to respond effectively to a clearly articulated problem.

Since the 1991 conference there has been increased and wide-spread concern and attention focused on the growth in racist activity, on the experiences of ethnic minorities in western Europe, and the involvement by young people in racist and extreme right-wing groups. What is also noticeable since the conference is the breaking of the taboo on discussing this major problem. The issue of racism and young people has now been recognized as one that requires increased understanding and vigilance.

However, what is also noticeable is the paucity of trans-European opportunities for youth workers and policy-makers to meet to share these concerns and examine how strategies can be used to counter racism. This book therefore is an attempt to move the debate on two levels. The first is to encourage and celebrate the diversity and difference in our multicultural/multiracial Europe. The second is to confront the development of negative thinking and racist activity among indigenous young people towards minorities living in their countries.

Explanation of terms

Before progressing further it is important to explain some of the main terms used in the book. As editors this provides us with a challenge, as racism, youth policy and youth work are understood differently in different countries.

(a) Racism

Racism has come to mean the domination of one group over another based on perceived racial differences. This implies that there is a hierarchical order in which certain groups of people are superior to others. For example, in The Netherlands, the Turks and the Moroccans occupy a position that is perceived as inferior

2

to the Surinamese. In turn the Surinamese are perceived as inferior to the indigenous Dutch population.

Even a cursory examination of a country's economic and social structure indicates that certain groups occupy positions above or below others. This is not an accident, but a social construction that has been arrived at over a number of years and is due to a series of social, cultural and political forces that have ascribed power to certain groups, leaving others powerless. Further analysis shows that there is a link in the way that colour, religion, cultural habits and geographical location have deemed groups of people as outsiders or insiders. The political, legal and social systems have legitimated and perpetuated these categorizations. The position of different groups in a country's hierarchical structure changes with national and international forces and in turn leads to the transformation of societies.

(b) Youth policy

All the countries discussed here have developed social policies as part of their delivery of welfare services. Traditionally, however, youth policy does not occupy a high profile within these social policies. With the fast-changing economic and social situation in Europe, countries have been keen to develop policies to incorporate and socialize young people who will participate in this new economic order. For example, in all European countries a great deal of energy and resources have been committed to vocational preparation and training of young people. Similarly, concerns over such issues as sexual health have led all European countries to develop health promotion policies and programmes targeted at young people.

While youth policy in Europe remains fragmented and diverse, it is developing in a way in which European Union countries are pooling their knowledge and expertise to form a more comprehensive approach to the problems facing their young people. The work by Cavalli & Galland (1995) is an attempt by academics to

3

analyse the trends affecting Europe's young people and the youth policy developments in selected countries. Furthermore the chapter by Lynne Chisholm in the Cavalli & Galland text demonstrates that the youth phase for all European young people has become extended, destandardized, fragmented and individualized. The force of this varies, however, from country to country. For example the participation rate in education varies across the European Union. In 1986–7, over 50 per cent of 15–19 year olds in the former FRG and Belgium were engaged in some form of part-time or full-time education/training. This compared with only 25 per cent of young people of the same age in the United Kingdom.

(c) Youth work

Youth work has developed in a disparate manner throughout Europe. Reflection on the history of youth work in different countries indicates a rich tradition much of which predates formal school education. In particular there was a good deal of work undertaken in working class neighbourhoods. Similarly, in most European countries the Church has been particularly involved in youth work prior to state involvement.

Although youth work is both diverse and different in the countries considered here, there are important similarities that give it its distinct and important position within the educational and welfare traditions. These are spelled out in more detail in each of the chapters. The main common themes are the voluntary relationship between youth worker and young person, the informal nature of the learning process, the opportunities for individual learning in the context of groups, and the use of a variety of creative activities to engage and involve young people. A central aspect of youth work in general is the participation of young people in decision-making processes in order to empower them. Youth work in the way described is, we believe, a valid activity for the strengthening and continuity of democracy. It also has an important role in celebrating cultural diversity and combating racism. Except in the chapter on Belgium youth work does not include youth organizations or youth movements.

(d) The countries selected

The countries chosen for examination reflect the diverse yet distinct nature of contemporary Europe. The *United Kingdom* and *The Netherlands* both have extensive histories as colonial powers and both have a long history of immigration. For example, post-war immigration to Britain commenced in the late 1940s and continued throughout the 1950s and 1960s before various immigration acts curtailed the influx of migrants from the new Commonwealth, in particular people from India, Pakistan, Bangladesh, the West Indies and East Africa.

Spain was chosen as it has traditionally been a country of emigration. In more recent times however, it has become a country of immigration with people settling from North Africa, and retired people from northern Europe, as well as Spaniards resettling in their country after living abroad.

Since 1945 *Germany* has experienced three kinds of immigration. The first group were the labour migrants who came after the Second World War from Yugoslavia, Greece, Turkey, Spain and North Africa. They assisted in the rebuilding of the German economy and occupied the unskilled sector of the labour market. As the German economy grew, and industry and commerce became increasingly automated, the need for such labour declined and migration was drastically reduced. The second wave of immigration came with people living in Eastern Europe whose families have German roots. These are the so-called *Aussiedlers*. After German reunification new tensions and problems developed in the integration of the disparate German identities. The third group of immigrants to Germany have been asylum seekers and refugees. While Germany has a traditionally lenient immigration policy towards those suffering persecution in their own countries this has changed in recent years with the German authorities greatly restricting entry to such people.

Belgium (Flanders) has been chosen for its uniqueness as a country that has transformed from a centralized to a federal state. This transformation has not been without its problems, particularly those relating to nationalism, and has led to the emergence of a number of extreme right-wing groups. The authors of the chapter on Belgium have focused their discussion on the Flanders region of the country, in which there has been a significant influx of north Africans.

Themes and approaches

When commissioning the chapters we asked the contributors to consider a range of themes that would provide a useful framework for contrasting and comparing each country. The themes the authors were requested to consider were:

- The social, economic and political background of the country.
- Useful data on the emigration/immigration affecting the country.
- The historical development and role of far-right extreme groupings.
- The country's social and youth policy.
- Relevant research on young people and race.
- The role of youth work and its relationship to anti-racist practice.

We were aware, however, that this framework could restrict discussion on important issues affecting young people in the countries selected. Contributors were therefore asked to use the framework only as a guide.

Nevertheless there are a number of important similarities among the countries. As noted above, although the debate on racism within particular countries has been evolving over several years, the discussion on a trans-European level is still in its infancy. What is worrying is that each country refuses to acknowledge in anything more than a superficial way its racist antecedents. We believe this is one of the major stumbling blocks to recognizing and dealing with racism in contemporary Europe. If greater acknowledgement and discussion had been accorded to recognizing Europe's racist roots we would be further along the line in tackling the racism we are witnessing in each of its countries. It has taken racist violence to alert Europe's liberal democracies to the seething undercurrent of racism. Perhaps if Europe had examined and learnt from its past we would not be in the situation we are currently facing.

Another common theme in the selected countries is the contradiction between restrictive immigration policies and social policy that attempts to integrate "foreigners" into the dominant culture. European governments' ambivalence towards foreigners has had a negative effect upon young people and has failed to provide them with a clear and uncontested view of a multicultural and multiracial society.

The various contributors' approaches reflect the different understanding of the challenges faced in their countries. In the first contribution, Keith Popple examines the United Kingdom's colonial past and its impact upon contemporary British life. Discussing the influence of the New Right he notes successive recent Conservative governments' regressive social policies and their failure to sign up to the Social Chapter at Maastricht. He then moves to demonstrate how racism has come to be exhibited in public policies and in the actions of young white people. The failure of the British government to present a positive position and action on racism means that a vacuum has been created, and this has been filled by extreme right-wing groupings. These are examined, as are the anti-racist movements which have attempted to win the attention and support of alienated young whites and young black people. On a micro-level he then considers how youth work has since the 1960s developed particular approaches that attempt to deal with the needs of young black people and with the reactions by young white people.

In the following chapter Yvonne Leeman and Sawitri Saharso examine The Netherlands' colonial past, its history of migrant labour and the impact upon the present composition of the population. Since the mid 1980s minority groups have grown in size and are now relatively evenly distributed throughout The Netherlands. The authors note that since 1983 the government has adopted an explicit minority policy focused upon integration. However, although a number of positive results have emanated from this policy, the majority of people from ethnic minorities continue to occupy low social and economic positions. To an extent this has been due to the recession and the restructuring of the labour market although, as the authors point out, a powerful force has been the nature and practice of racism. Leeman & Saharso discuss how racism came to be explicitly presented on the political scene through the founding, in 1971, of the NVU (Dutch People's Union). Since then the image of The Netherlands as a tolerant society has been damaged by a series of racial incidents.

In the latter part of their chapter the contributors examine how racism is challenged both in the outlawing of racist activity and in the implementation of policies aimed at promoting multi-ethnic participation. On a national level this policy has been translated into the distribution of information, while examples are provided of local projects that reflect successful work. In general, the authors conclude, there is a lack of knowledge and experience of methods that can be used to interest and influence young people in the area of anti-racism and tolerance.

In the next contribution Pablo Angel Meira Cartea and José Antonio Caride Gómez begin by describing the historical background of Spain's immigrant population which up to now has been relatively small. The economic crisis of the 1970s propelled western European countries to adopt restrictive immigration policies and led to Spain's southern coastline becoming known as the "frontier of Europe". At the same time Spain introduced strict immigration controls on people coming from third world countries. Although Spain has a long tradition of racist attitudes towards gypsies, its self-image has been one of a non-racist country with none of the major political parties supporting a racist ideology. Although discrimination against minority groups was made illegal in 1985, there has been a growth in racist activity since that date.

While the authors argue that both legislation and the social and economic initiatives relating to immigration are far from desirable they point to positive measures being taken to confront racism. They discuss the plan presented by the Spanish Council of Ministers in which they hope to counter socio-political and economic inequality by working with young people through associations and youth councils. The contributors describe the collective work during the first half of the 1990s to promote welfare and integrate adolescents from ethnic minorities into mainstream Spanish society. This approach has been two-pronged: first, to provide schooling for gypsy children, and second to design and deliver preventive measures to counter discrimination against young people because of their ethnicity or religion.

In the next contribution Rudolf Leiprecht, Lena Inowlocki, Athanasios Marvakis and Jürgen Novak indicate that discussions focusing on racism are new in Germany. The authors begin by comparing Germany's reputation for responding positively to millions of fellow Germans and economic refugees directly after the Second World War with its recent hostility towards immigrants. Ethnic inequality can be seen in minorities' lack of political expression and in their unequal legal status.

Next, the authors examine the historical differences of both the Germanys – the old FRG and GDR – as well as the effect of national sentiment on the risk of the formation of extreme right-wing groups. They discuss modernization theory and question its explanation of the emergence of right-wing thinking and acting. They shed new light on the role of gender in regard to racial violence, arguing that both men and women are engaged in violent activity towards people from ethnic minorities. Finally, they discuss different approaches to handling racism in youth work in which controversial, so-called acceptance youth work is highlighted. They end by stressing the importance of understanding racism and anti-racism as ways of thinking that relate to specific situations rather than to particular aspects of a human being.

In the final chapter Danny Wildemeersch and Gie Redig examine the political scene of Flanders, which together with the Walloon and Brussels regions make up the federalization of Belgium. Since the mid 1970s racism has become more apparent and is now established in the political party, the Flemish Bloc, which has shifted its previous nationalist bias to its present racist position. At the same time there has been a general and growing intolerance shown by the Flemish population towards foreigners who are not integrated into Flemish institutions and social life. Wildemeersch and Redig argue that this is a characteristic of Flanders as a dual society.

The authors describe ways in which politicians representing the federal and the regional levels have now taken a stand against racism. In 1989 the Royal Commissioner for Migrant Affairs was appointed and introduced the notion of "insertion" of minorities in society. This notion was accepted and adopted by the Belgian parliament and has since been its policy towards the migrant population. Youth work is considered a powerful resource for promoting the social integration of young people from migrant groups. At the same time the authors recognize the role youth work has in challenging racism.

Finally, Wildemeersch and Redig conclude with a discussion of five examples of Flemish youth work that, on a modest scale, are attempting to overcome the dualistic tendencies in their society.

Racism in youth policy and youth work: the need for challenge and change

It will be seen from the following chapters that racism is the norm in European countries. Although reflected in individuals' actions and words, racism is not a matter of a few people's behaviour. To concentrate on the local and the individual disregards the role of institutional racism and fails to account for indirect or unintentional racism. Such a view ignores the often subtle racism of the majority, it pathologizes the few noisy overt racists, and it avoids examination of the links between structural forces and individuals' behaviour.

Racism is basically a form of social control. It functions to ration resources and keeps in place a social and economic hierarchy that benefits from its existence and perpetuation. Racism operates to the advantage of the few, while enslaving the majority. Everyone has everything to gain from celebrating the diversity of modern Europe, and everything to gain from challenging racism. Ultimately, European governments need to devise and introduce policies covering labour, income and housing in order to protect ethnic minorities. In turn, youth policy, and especially youth work, can make an important contribution to promote intercultural learning and understanding. At the same time, we believe youth policy and youth work need to adopt anti-racist policies and practice to assist in transforming the present worrying trends emerging in our midst. If this is to succeed there is a great need to pool our ideas and experiences. The following contributions are part of this important and timely debate.

Reference

Cavalli, A. & O. Galland (eds) 1995. *Youth in Europe: social change in Western Europe*. London: Pinter.

11

2
—

Understanding and tackling racism among young people in the United Kingdom

Keith Popple

Introduction

In order that we can critically review the recent policy and practice developments that have been implemented to challenge racism amongst Britain's young people, we need first to examine the macro setting in which this has taken place. Our discussion will therefore commence by exploring the contemporary social, economic and political scene in the UK. We will then move to specifically consider the area of "race", including the rise and role of far-right and fascist groups and the response by anti-racist groups. The discussion will continue by focusing on youth policy and youth work in the UK before examining the strategies that have been deployed to address the issue of "race" and racism. Finally, the chapter will assess what this means in practice.

The United Kingdom today

The most prominent feature of contemporary UK economic, social and political life has been the influence of Thatcherite or New Right policies. Named after the British Conservative Prime

Minister (1979–90) Margaret Thatcher, Thatcherism has come to mean the primacy of wealth creation; the regulation of distribution through market principles, accompanied by the notion of individual rather than public choice; redistribution based upon the theory of "trickle down"; an attack on, and a restructuring of, large areas of public and private activity; an assault on the influence of the trade union movement; and the notion of poverty as being absolute as opposed to relative. The Conservatives did not, however, perform the economic miracle they promised and the rise of the New Right was accompanied by an economic recession borne disproportionately by the poor. Statistics for 1991–92 show that real disposable income, that is cash left over after taxes, National Insurance and pension contributions, was almost 80 per cent higher than in 1971. However, the increasing wealth is far from evenly distributed. The share of income for the poorest fifth of the population had fallen from 10 per cent when the Conservatives took power in 1979, to 6 per cent in 1990–91. In contrast over the same period, the richest fifth of the population had increased its share of wealth from 35 per cent to 43 per cent (Central Statistical Office 1991).

The increasing divide between the rich and the poor in the UK has also been reflected in the unemployment rate. In January 1997 Britain's official unemployment rate stood at just under 2 million. However, it has been estimated by the Unemployment Unit that the 30 changes in the methods of counting unemployed people since 1979 have disguised a much higher figure of about 1 million more people (Unemployment Unit and Youth Aid 1990). Unemployment is, however, not random. People's age, gender, occupation and race are all features in the shaping of unemployment. For instance, in the years 1987 to 1989 the unemployment rate for young people from minority ethnic groups was almost double that for the young white population. 21 per cent of the minority ethnic 16–24 age groups were unemployed compared with 12 per cent of whites of the same age. There are differences within minority ethnic groups with 27 per cent of Pakistanis and Bangladeshis unemployed and 25 per cent from the West Indian/

Guyanese group (Department of Employment 1991). The increasing divide between people is also demonstrated in occupation categories. Women, for example, are over-represented in low-paid work, part-time work, and in work that is either temporary, seasonal or casual.

A feature of recent political life in Britain has been the discussion of whether to participate fully in the European Union. This was brought to a head in the House of Commons debate on the Maastricht treaty during the summer of 1993. Although the United Kingdom is a full Member State of the European Union it is the only Member State not to sign the Charter of the Fundamental Social Rights of Workers. This means that while the United Kingdom enjoys the benefits of strengthened European co-operation its citizens will not be covered by the progressive social policy the EU is attempting to develop.

"Race" in Britain

(a) Immigration and settlement

The issue of "race" has always been high on the UK political and social agenda. The focus for this is directly linked to the country's former large and sprawling Empire in which, at one time, all its peoples were subjects of the British Crown. Soon after the end of the Second World War, the British government and many large British companies encouraged certain groups of people from the colonies to move to the UK to work in the newly expanding public services, and in the industrial and service sectors. On entry most of the immigrants found themselves working in the least well-paid and the dirtiest jobs, and residing in the worst housing. The influx of newcomers was, however, to spark a degree of unrest when the indigenous white Britons believed their employment prospects could be threatened. In 1958 there were attacks on West Indian people and homes in both Notting Hill in London,

15

and in the city of Nottingham. The Conservative government, sensitive to a white backlash, and concerned that it could lose votes and seats at the next general election, introduced the 1962 Commonwealth Immigrants Act, which restricted the number of black people coming into Britain. This Act was the first of many passed by both Conservative and Labour governments in an attempt to control the influx of black people.

While the 1962 and 1968 Commonwealth Immigrants Acts, the 1969 Immigration Appeals Act and the 1971 Immigration Act restricted immigration, the 1965 and 1968 Race Relations Acts took the first steps towards outlawing discrimination and establishing the Community Relations Commission (which later became the Commission for Racial Equality). The government was in effect signalling a mixed message. On the one hand it was claiming, by restricting entry, that black people were a problem, while on the other hand they were advocating that the indigenous population should welcome the new settlers.

Moving to contemporary times we note that the 1991 UK Population Census reveals that 5.5 per cent of the total population is non-white (HMSO 1993a). In Greater London, which has a population of nearly 7 million people, the non-white population is 20.2 per cent (HMSO 1993b). These and other figures on minority ethnic groups provide us with up-to-date and accurate data that can play an important role in identifying patterns of disadvantage and the various processes that produce them. We have seen above that black people are more likely to be unemployed than whites. We also know that although black people account for 5.5 per cent of the population they make up 15 per cent of the prison population of England and Wales (Central Statistical Office 1991). Burns (1990) has reported that an estimated 63 per cent of young black people experience some adversarial contact with the police, compared with 35 per cent of white people of the same age. The same report also reveals that about one in ten black males are likely to be imprisoned by the time they are twenty-one years of age. One of the reasons for this situation is racism within the police force. For example, in 1989 the Gifford

Report examined the extent of racism in Liverpool, particularly within its police force. The Report concluded that there was a wholly unacceptable level of racist language and racist behaviour by officers of rank in the Merseyside Force (The Gifford Report July 1989, quoted in the *Independent* 19 August 1989).

If we examine statistics related to the racial origin of crime victims we find that black people of Afro-Caribbean and Asian origin tend to be more at risk from a whole range of crime than white people. The work by Mayhew et al. (1989) also finds that black people have less confidence in the police response to their need for assistance.

We have noted above the development of racist feelings towards black people in Britain. Many of these feelings have been translated into racist jokes, behaviour, language and attitudes. There have also been racially motivated incidents and attacks on black people. In 1988 4,383 racial incidents were reported to the police. Four years later in 1992 the figure was 7,734 (Home Office 1993). The Home Office does not keep a record of the seriousness of incidents, which can range from violent attacks to verbal abuse. Whether there has been a real increase in incidents is uncertain as the black community have traditionally been suspicious of the police and have almost certainly under-reported incidents in the past. The rise may in part be due therefore to an increase in the confidence of victims and in the ability and willingness of the police to assist.

It would of course be unwise to believe that all British people are engaged in overt racist acts. This is plainly not the case. What is indisputable is that white Britons as a group have benefited from racism. One only has to look at the key social policy areas to see the way in which black people are disadvantaged. For example in housing we find evidence of differential housing outcomes for minority ethnic groups. This has been summarized in the following way:

> In the 1980s then, the NCWP[1] minorities still live in significantly worse quality housing and in poorer, less popu-

lar areas than the white British population. This holds across and within all tenures. Indeed, the high level of owner occupation amongst Asians (72 per cent as against 59 per cent of the general population) provides no guarantee of good housing . . . the prevailing trend in many cities over the last two decades has been one of growing residential segregation between NCWP minorities and whites, with the former becoming increasingly over-represented in the poorest areas (Phillips 1987: 108).

Similarly, in the area of health we find a high degree of discriminatory practice. The National Health Service has for many years employed minority ethnic people but examination of the data shows they are concentrated in ancillary jobs, for example in domestic, catering, cleaning and maintenance services (CRE 1983). A later study demonstrates that minority ethnic National Health Service doctors were located in less popular and low status jobs, for example in geriatrics and psychiatry. Furthermore, the research found that 50 per cent of "non-white" doctors and 40 per cent of their white colleagues believed there was racial discrimination in the National Health Service (CRE 1987).

Perhaps the most disturbing feature of the overt racism in Britain has been the recent resurgence of racist and fascist groups that we now examine.

(b) Organized racist and fascist activity

At the present time there are four significant ultra-right-wing movements in the UK: the National Front; the British Movement; Combat 18; and the British National Party. Each grouping has fostered racial hatred and violence and inspired fascist thuggery. The most prominent of these organizations is the British National Party (BNP).

Developing rapidly since the mid-1980s the BNP has a national membership of around 2,000. This is supplemented by some

10,000 members and supporters of the skinhead Nazi "Blood and Honour" group which is now under BNP control (Platt 1992). According to Ford (1992) the leaders of the increasingly active BNP have serious criminal convictions ranging from organizing illegal paramilitary groups, possession of firearms and the making of bombs, to a number of convictions centred on race relations and public order. The BNP sees one of its key roles as influencing young people and much of its racist material is directed at school students and the young unemployed. It has a strategy of "educating" the young with a range of racist and anti-Semitic books, videos and audio tapes, which are sold through a book club, thereby avoiding prosecution under the law. The BNP also publishes a monthly magazine called *Spearhead* and *British Nationalist*, a monthly newspaper. Both are sold in public places, often where young people (particularly males) meet, for instance outside football league grounds on match days.

Like other racist and fascist movements the BNP has tapped into young people's fears and anxieties for their future. We have noted above the contemporary economic difficulties that the UK is experiencing. These are likely to remain in the foreseeable future, and with young people continuing to face problems in obtaining worthwhile and well-paid employment, they are increasingly likely to look for political explanations of their predicament. In the face of economic deprivation, and the failure of mainstream political parties to respond effectively to the problem, the BNP provides a simple and apparently logical explanation. "Get rid of the blacks and the Jews and you will be better off." To quote Ray Hill, a fascist turned anti-fascist,

> I became a fascist because the fascists got there first . . . It acts as a magnet to many rebellious and disaffected white youths who see everything they are interested in, from football matches to raves, criminalised by the state and derided by many in the middle class. The youth who join the fascist movement are as much victims of its ideology as those they persecute, because they are used by the

middle-class leadership and will either end up in jail or with poisoned minds (*The Guardian* 1994).

In September 1993 the BNP won its first ever local election seat, only to lose it at the election in the following May. It is uncertain whether the BNP will succeed in winning any further seats although what is clear is that it will continue in its attempts to win over the hearts and minds of the disillusioned young white people living in the poorest areas of Britain. We also know there has been a sharp increase in racially motivated attacks with the BNP keeping up its pressure on black people. According to Platt (1992) when the BNP established its headquarters at Welling, South London, there was a 140 per cent increase in racial attacks in the area. In July 1995 the local council ruled that the head-quarters should be closed.

In 1992 a small non-hierarchical group calling itself Combat 18 (C18) split from the BNP. An internal document by C18 reveals a hard-line group disaffected with democratic politics and the failure of legal fascist parties to win electoral support. Instead, C18 advocate tactics of violence and, in the document, explain how to attack non-whites and provoke racial conflict. C18 have been active in leading disorder at international football matches involving England and The Netherlands (in 1993), and England and Ireland (in 1995).

In response to the growing number of attacks upon black people, and the increased activity of the racist and fascist movements, the Anti-Nazi League, which was active in the 1970s, was relaunched in January 1992. Two months earlier the Anti-Racist Alliance was formed. Both movements, which have attracted a large participation by young people, are engaged in the struggle to confront the racist movements. A further small grouping engaged in direct action, including violence, is Anti-Fascist Action.

(c) Anti-racist movements

(i) The Anti-Nazi League (ANL)

The ANL emerged as a national social movement in 1977 in response to the increased activity of the fascist National Front among young people. Although the ANL drew its support from different age groups it was particularly attractive to young people. The Rock Against Racism campaign launched by the ANL increased its popular appeal among sections of the working class youth that were likely to be attracted to the National Front. With the decline of the National Front as a political force from 1979, the ANL's activity similarly decreased. The growth of racist and fascist movements in the UK in the early 1990s, and in particular the BNP's attacks on black communities, led to the relaunch of the ANL.

The relaunched ANL combines a range of black and left-activist groupings. A number of anti-racists have argued that the new ANL is similar to its predecessor and is a front for the Trotskyite Socialist Worker Party which has a tradition of involving itself in popular struggles as a method of recruiting members and influencing events. Certainly a central strategy is to confront racists and fascists on the streets. This is colloquially called "Bashing the Fash". By adopting this approach the ANL believes it can eradicate the "Fash" while uniting black and white people. This strategy has led to a certain amount of disagreement and jostling with the Anti-Racist Alliance.

(ii) The Anti-Racist Alliance (ARA)

The ARA was formed in November 1991 mainly by former black activists who had been working in the Labour Party. Its organizers claim it is the sole black-led anti-racist movement. They argue that black self-organization together with support from the Labour Party, trade unions and black community groups is the only way to combat racism. The key strategy of the ARA is to urge the government to introduce legislation making racial

21

harassment a specific offence and prevent the sale or distribution of racist literature. The ARA argue that confronting fascists and racists in the manner advocated by the ANL is counterproductive. They believe such activity achieves little in combating racism. It may grab the headlines and embarrass the right, but the racists continue to campaign and it is local black people who suffer the backlash from racists in the area (*The Guardian* 1993).

A further complaint from the ARA about the ANL's tactics is that its focus on far-right groups ignores issues such as state racism and the threat to minority ethnic groups in the European Union (Platt 1992).

(iii) The Anti-Fascist Action (AFA)

The AFA is a small, clandestine nationwide organization established in 1985 by former ANL supporters. It has a policy of confronting the far-right both ideologically and physically. Most of its members come from the same constituency that the BNP tries to recruit from: white working-class young people from depressed areas that have a high proportion of black people. The AFA has been criticized by other anti-racist organizations and targeted by the police for its violence. AFA supporters claim however, that its tactics have worked and kept fascist groups in check.

We can see that the economic problems in the UK have become a breeding ground for a certain number of the disillusioned young white people who face a bleak future. The position for young black people is even worse, and yet as we have noted they are likely to be the convenient scapegoat in the deteriorating situation. The growth of racist and fascist movements, and in particular the BNP, is of concern as they are targeting their vile literature at arguably the most vulnerable young whites. The BNP has also been engaged in racist attacks, providing young white people, and in particular young white males, with an outlet for their pent-up misplaced anger and resentment.

With the situation facing young British white and black people outlined, we move to consider what has been undertaken in the area of youth policy and youth work to combat racism.

Youth policy and youth work

In the UK social policy has come to mean the political, economic, sociological and socio-legal examination of the ways in which central and local government policies affect communities and individuals. The main areas of social policy cover education, housing, health, social security, personal social services, criminal justice and, increasingly, employment and training. At present youth policy does not exist as a discrete area. Instead it is a field of study within social policy that examines the impact of a range of policies on the young. The main areas of social policy that affect young people are education policy, juvenile justice, and vocational preparation and training. In recent years there has been an increase in health policy initiatives that have targeted young people, the most prominent of which have related to educating young people about the dangers of smoking and the health risks attached to certain sexual behaviour. Similarly in the last ten years policies within the areas of social security and housing have affected many young people.

Although historically it appears that social policies affecting young people have developed in a fragmented manner Davies (1986) argues that since the mid 1970s youth policy has emerged within a coherent framework that serves the government's economic and political concerns. Davies's view is that the New Right have successfully harnessed the public's fear of youth (hence the double-edged title of his book, *Threatening Youth*) with legislation that has defined and structured young people's position within society. The state has intervened in such a way as to undermine the power and influence of professionals running services for young people by locating more power and responsibility in agencies that have followed the new hard-nosed government policies, and by financially restructuring services. Youth work is one area of state provision that has been restructured and where expenditure has been reduced.

1944

1960

Although youth work has existed in the UK in one form or another since the nineteenth century it was not until the passing of the 1944 Education Act that it was recognized as an activity that warranted state finance and support. It was given a significant boost with the publication of the Albermarle Report (HMSO 1960) which highlighted the inadequacy of the existing provision and led to an expansion of youth work in youth clubs and youth centres. The situation now is diverse with some youth clubs and centres operated by local authorities and others by voluntary organizations. Some of these clubs and centres are well resourced and are open several nights a week while the majority of clubs, especially those run by voluntary organizations, are open only once or twice a week. The quality of premises used by these clubs is variable, ranging from village halls to purpose-built centres. Many youth workers are engaged in work with young people in places other than centres and clubs. For instance detached workers meet young people in coffee bars, cafes and city centres. Although the majority of youth workers are part-time, either paid or volunteers, it has been estimated that there are around 4,900 full-time youth workers employed by local authorities and voluntary organizations.

Traditional leisure-based youth work focusing upon the social education needs of young people, as developed within the Youth Service in England and Wales, has, as indicated, suffered from a drastic reduction in its funding in the last two decades. At the same time young people in their mid and late teenage years are increasingly rejecting the often unexciting and paternalistic youth clubs for more attractive commercial provision. They are also more likely than their predecessors to be enjoying home leisure activities such as video games and computer technology. An important article on the changing structure and content of youth work and the Youth Service has argued that large-scale changes are affecting the shape of the activity (Jeffs & Smith 1990). The authors argue that the reduction in local authority functions, power and resources will lead to central government deciding on priorities for publicly funded youth work. Similarly within local authorities a number of departments will compete between themselves and with other agencies, such as the police, for funds that would previously been the Youth Service's.

Youth work has then undergone a major change in the last few years. Although work in clubs still forms the bulk of the activity there is an increasing amount of work targeted at particular groups and around specific issues. At the same time, practitioners are to be found in a range of disciplines and organizations outside of the statutory and voluntary youth work sectors. There is, for example, a good deal of youth work directed around the issues of drug and alcohol abuse, with young people who are unable to find satisfactory living accommodation, and work focused on the issue of juvenile crime.

However, youth work that is funded exhibits four general yet central features that distinguish the work from other interventions with the young. One is the primacy of the voluntary element. Generally, the relationship between the youth worker and the young person is a voluntary one. This is unlike the mandatory relationship between teacher and pupil. The second feature is the informal and non-prescriptive nature of the work. The third feature is the scope for young people to choose their own point of contact, for example through outreach work and detached work, which is outside of formal institutions. The final feature is that youth work, unlike a great deal of other provision for the young, is not engaged in offering young people formal qualifications. The unique setting in which youth work is practised therefore provides valuable opportunities and a potentially receptive environment in which to challenge racism.

Informality and non-prescriptive nature of the work viewed as a 'potentially receptive environment' for countering racism (Popple 1997: 25)

Educational approaches to tackling racism

Since the 1960s a number of educational approaches have been used in youth work to tackle racism. Reviewing these approaches it is possible to identify four major categories: monocultural, multicultural, anti-racist, and cultural and political approaches. As we will see these approaches reflect specific ideas and the different periods in which they evolved. Consideration is now made of these.

(a) Monocultural approaches

Monocultural educational approaches aim to encourage people living in the UK to view themselves as British citizens. In this sense all citizens are expected to adopt the social and cultural practices and habits of the host society. Monocultural education strategies developed in the 1950s and 1960s as a response to the numerically significant post-war black immigration into the UK. This post-war immigration from the black Commonwealth was encouraged by the government because of Britain's labour shortage problems. The general assumption was that black people settling in the UK had few requirements, and in so far as they did then these would be met as soon as they were assimilated. Black people were encouraged to believe they should be grateful for a place within British society and in return become model citizens by adopting British culture. This is in itself problematic as the terms "British" and "culture" have debatable and contested meanings. The belief was that by black people adopting such a stance they could more easily assimilate and integrate into British society, so reducing racial hatred. This process has been described in the following way. The migrants gradually learn to "adapt" to the values and expectations of the host culture and for their part the hosts slowly "accept" the migrants as permanent members of society. As migrants – or their descendants – are socialized into the dominant values, and misunderstandings are

EDUCATIONAL APPROACHES TO TACKLING RACISM

increasingly resolved, so the newcomers are increasingly incorporated into the over-arching consensus (Richardson & Lambert 1985: 30).

The assumption central to monocultural approaches is that minority ethnic groups should adapt and change, relinquishing their "alien" cultures in order to be assimilated into the host society. The anticipated adjustment is, in essence, one-way and underestimates black people's wish to maintain their own cultures. This approach has been described as a "colour-blind approach" (Dominelli 1988). The "colour-blind approach" was typical of the line taken in the Albemarle Report (HMSO 1960), which offered a limited analysis of the need for youth work either to confront racism or to respond to the issues faced by young black people. This was in spite of riots and street battles in 1958, mentioned previously. An example of the Report's limited understanding is reflected in the following extract.

> It is also important to recognise that in many industrial towns the areas with sub-standard housing are undergoing fundamental social changes that have sometimes led to serious disturbances among some of the young people. New and strange faces appear on the doorsteps and congregate in the streets as workers from many lands find a job and a home in Britain. The integration of these families brings problems, and has sometimes created a sense of insecurity and a fear among the established community that housing standards will deteriorate further. Housing conditions do not completely explain the violence shown by some youths in these areas, and the prevalence of lawless gangs is not a new social phenomenon of the slums. However these racial outbursts present a new problem and seem paradoxical in this age when young people of all races and nationalities seem less different and share common interests such as jazz and football and often a common culture (HMSO 1960: 19–20).

27

Nearly forty years later this statement, which draws a causal link between black people and the decline in housing standards, and expresses surprise at the outburst of racial conflict, appears naive and ill-informed.

Subsequent reports, most notably the Hunt Report (DES 1967), the Fairbairn-Milson Report (DES 1969), and the work by Hartley (1971), argue that the Youth Service could assist in the absorption of young migrants into British society. The Hunt Report, for example, which was compiled when some one million black people were living in the UK, argues that racial harmony could be achieved by encouraging black and white young people to use the same youth clubs. The Report argues that urgent steps had to be undertaken to avoid racial strife. To quote the Hunt Report, "If England is not be the scene of race riots then the time for action is now. Tomorrow is too late" (DES 1967: 36).

The Fairbairn-Milson Report endorsed the findings of the Hunt Report recommending their implementation in the Youth Service. It also recommended that school buildings should be made available for community use in areas where black people were living. Furthermore the Fairbairn-Milson Report recommended that the needs of young black people should be kept under continuous review with local authorities working in conjunction with Community Relations Councils to assist with information, advice, training and conferences. Neither the Hunt Report, the Fairbairn-Milson Report, nor the work by Hartley recognized the particular needs of black young people or the negative impact of racism on their lives. All three were concerned instead with racial harmony.

In time, it became clear that monocultural strategies were having no real impact in absorbing black people into British life, while the positive contribution of minority ethnic cultures to the country's economic, cultural and social life were being overlooked. The outcome in the 1970s was the emergence of multicultural approaches to education.

28

(b) Multicultural approaches

Multicultural approaches both celebrate and attempt to protect and stress the importance of cultural variety within society. The purpose is to encourage tolerance, respect and understanding of minority cultures. Unlike monocultural approaches, which assert that "everyone is the same and should be treated the same", multicultural perspectives claim to respond to the *"individual* needs of everyone".

There are a number of critics of multicultural approaches. Black writers in particular have argued that multiculturism does not address the basic power relationships inherent in racism. Bhavnani (1986) for example, argues that such approaches, with their preoccupation with cultural difference, has led to a concentration upon the exotic and unusual. The result, she argues, is an approach that is patronizing and offensive, reinforcing the stereotypical racist images of "alien" cultures. Other critics (Cole 1989; Troyna & Williams 1986) have attacked multiculturalism as focusing on the cultural differences between black and white people. Multicultural education therefore becomes a "saris, steel bands and samosas" approach, reducing an examination of black culture to a superficial level. In this perspective racism is an attitudinal problem. It does not, according to its critics, discuss the social and economic structures that both unite and separate people. Critics also see multiculturalism as strengthening racism by providing black people with positive self-images that serve to placate and dilute their demands while allowing the insidious effect of racism to continue (Sivanandan 1990). What is important for critics like Sivanandan is to view other cultures from a objective position. "Just to learn about other people's cultures is not to learn about the racism of one's own. To learn about the racism of one's own culture, on the other hand, is to approach other cultures objectively" (Sivanandan 1983: 5).

The moves towards multicultural approaches were reflected in the Youth Service, which itself is firmly rooted in the British education system. Two important reports published at the end of the

1970s reflect this perspective. One was the Community Relations Commission's study (CRC 1977) which discovered that although about 33 per cent of black young people had attended youth clubs, only 10 per cent were continuing to attend at the time of the fieldwork. The study also found that Asians were less likely to use youth clubs and centres than either Afro-Caribbean or Cypriot young people. It concluded that the Hunt Committee's recommendations were being interpreted in an uncritical manner with little evidence of multiracial provision. The other significant report, produced three years later (CRE 1980), warned of the problems that were being stored up by not addressing the needs of black young people. This was to prove insightful and the following year street riots involving both white and black young people took place in a number of British cities. Although these two reports had moved to acknowledge the presence of racism, they failed to address its structural roots. So while there was increased awareness of young black people's needs, for example their demand for separate provision, there was a tendency to promote youth activity which was thought beneficial to community relations. The outcome was events such as cultural evenings, rather than activities requested by young black people. There has therefore been some question as to whether multicultural approaches in youth work benefit anyone. Chauhan (1990) has argued that the approaches neither effectively challenge racism nor meet black people's needs.

In the early 1980s, with Thatcherism getting into its stride, public services were reviewed by the government with the aim of making them more efficient and effective. Youth work did not escape this examination, and a committee chaired by Alan Thompson, a retired civil servant, was established to consider the scope and content of the Youth Service in England and Wales. The resultant Thompson Report (HMSO 1982) identified three significant issues that affected contemporary young people: unemployment, racism and homelessness. Regarding racism the Report made three main recommendations. The first urged the need to respond fully to the needs of black young people. The

Meet needs, promote equality, involve people.

second recommended the lobbying and implementation of equal opportunity policies. Lastly, a recommendation was made that the black community should participate in the content, staffing, delivery and direction of the Youth Service. These recommendations signalled a positive shift in the understanding of young black people's needs and received support from a number of practitioners and policy-makers. The Thompson Report stated that youth provision should reflect the values and attitudes of the neighbourhoods where young people belong. This can lead to both specific and separate clubs for black young people, while encouraging the use of provision by all young people, irrespective of their cultural and ethnic background.

+ve report but never implemented across the country.

(c) Anti-racist approaches

Municipal

Guine 2000 has argued there only had a two year implementation.

In recent years new and important educational approaches have evolved to tackle racism in the UK. These anti-racist approaches argue that we live in an unequal society in which a complex range of inequalities including class, "race", gender, age, and disability operate to divide and contain people. This argument continues that it is impossible to deal with "race" or racism in isolation from the wider political, economic and social processes that over time have served to institutionalize power inequality. There has been a considerable debate centred on the issue of anti-racist strategies and multicultural approaches and the differences between the two. The distinction between the models has been described by Cohen. The liberal or multicultural position rightly resists the compulsory morality of "positive images" but fails to recognize the forms of hidden persuasion that exist in the education system and the wider society. Anti-racists are much better at highlighting these dimensions of hegemony, but if they use the most sophisticated theoretical work to expose the hidden ideological manoeuvres of racism, they no less strenuously exempt their own practices of propaganda from similar critical scrutiny (Cohen 1988: 96).

1993 Rywdt SCt dont plus other repts hylyht this facture of leaderstp

several problems with this approach

Bennett: 2000

No critical self reflection

Essentialising tendencies

31

A number of writers place multicultural approaches at the other end of a continuum from anti-racist approaches. For example, Grinter (1985) has argued that multiculturalists seek reforms within existing structures, whereas anti-racists seek to transform them. Troyna (1987) has commented that this is an oversimplified picture. "Closer scrutiny of the themes and concerns of anti-racist educational policy statements reveals a continuity and communality with earlier multicultural imperatives" (Troyna 1987: 7).

Parekh (1986), who advocates multicultural approaches, has criticized anti-racist approaches as being synonymous with anti-racist propaganda which in his view is little different from more progressive multicultural perspectives. Todd (1991) states that although the arguments surrounding multiculturalism and anti-racism assist in the clarification of the conceptual basis of educational methods, they are also unhelpful because the debate between the two has become insular and self-perpetuating. Todd (1991) and other writers, such as Leicester (1986) and Craft & Klein (1986), believe that successful anti-racist practice must synthesize the two. This is described in the following way.

> The polarisation in current literature of "multi-culturalists" as simply concerned with diversity, and "anti-racist" as concerned with the struggle for equality, is not helpful; these are not polar opposites; they share a complex inter-relationship . . . [they are] not alternatives, but interlocking parts of one whole, each is essential, but neither is sufficient on its own (Craft & Klein 1986: 42).

Cohen believes one way forward is to connect that which is progressive in both anti-racist and multicultural approaches with what might be described as a cultural approach. This synthesis takes popular culture and the way different groups of people see and understand the world as its starting point. This approach is similar to that described in Smith's (1988) advocacy of informal education, mutual aid and popular practice within youth work (see also Jeffs & Smith 1989).

[Handwritten margin note, left:] Draw on Yaa Asare's work Runnymede Trust 2009 + T. Troyna

[Handwritten margin note, bottom left:] Fits with youth work practice of listening to young people.

Synthesise Anti racism with multi culturalism and stress interconnected nni of oppression

(iv) Cultural and political approaches

Another productive way forward is to link young people's cultural milieu with a political understanding and form cultural and political approaches which recognize that individual attitudes and behaviour occur within a framework defined by the wider economic, political and social forces within society. This in turn provides opportunities to make connections between institutional discriminations and "race", gender and class inequalities (see Popple 1990). Cultural and political approaches attempt to build on the common experiences of disadvantage shared by black and white young people alike, for example by exploring together the problems of finding suitable affordable housing, of coping with unemployment or low income, of poor educational opportunities and reduced welfare and health services. These approaches are primarily processes whereby young people can begin to understand the complex relationships that shape their lives and how both black and white young people have similar but different experiences that determine their futures.

In an article that explores the possibilities for anti-racist strategies in white working-class areas, Warren (1990) posits a similar view. He stresses the need for committed youth workers to work from an experimental, non-prescriptive and anti-oppressive perspective where they work alongside young people, rather than encouraging them to uncritically accept society's prevailing attitudes. The British state, claims Warren, is capitalist, imperialist and patriarchal and therefore resistance has to be "centred around the analysis of common experience and juxtaposed against such prevalent ideologies to render visible that which is artificial" (Warren 1990: 7). It is only in this way that racism, sexism and classism will be confronted and undermined. Using an example of the school system Warren reflects how it operates against the interests of working-class young people so that as adults they control little power in the economic, social and political spheres. This disadvantage can lead them to become distanced from more privileged sectors of society and create

maintain a focus on racism — *Does not* *stays surface on white-world.* *pg 6*

ghetto-like communities which, because of their powerlessness, are easily controlled by the criminal justice system should they protest against their situation. Warren believes youth workers are in a unique position to highlight for young people a whole range of disadvantages and draw analogies between the positions that both black and white young people find themselves occupying. Such approaches can, he argues, assist them to question how much affinity either group has with so-called British culture. Youth workers can explore with young people what British ideology serves to protect and expose it as both classist and racist. Once this common experience is identified and explored, Warren asserts, false ideologies can be exploded and the futility of discriminating on grounds of colour finally recognized.

As we have noted, cultural and political approaches are distinguished by their view that racism is an integral part of a number of interlinked forms of oppression and inequality. Rather than attempting to change individual behaviour, cultural and political approaches offer opportunities for black and white young people to identify similarities in their situations and the forces that determine their position within a hierarchically structured society. When awareness is raised scope exists for more fully motivated support against racism; for example within whole communities, or within more broadly conceived equal opportunities initiatives.

The way forward?

We have discussed above the different educational approaches developed to tackle racism in the UK, and how they have been adapted for use in youth work. One of the main drawbacks to the more radical approaches, such as anti-racist and cultural and political approaches, is the resistance to them from powerful groups within society. By their very nature such educational approaches question and challenge the status quo and are therefore unlikely to be validated and resourced by those who are

34

Gaine's model of PCS — see also Thompson.
Danemark's stratified ontology.

potentially threatened by the practice and policy outcomes. It seems improbable that clear anti-racist policy directives and strategies will be formulated and implemented on a national level when central government opinion has openly attacked anti-racist discourse. Furthermore, it is questionable whether educational approaches within youth work will make a significant difference to the fight against racism. The implementation of radical approaches at the micro level raises consciousness among those with little power to use it. The most effective change is likely to be that which takes place at the macro level.

Need sequential

Macro + Micro stratified required.

It is highly unlikely that radical change will ever be brought about by a sense of charitable or moral concern for the plight of minority ethnic groups in the UK. Whether one supports the notion of a narrow power elite, a plural elite or a diffused power structure, it is apparent that Britain's social and economic system is constructed to benefit those who hold power. Those who occupy these pivotal positions of power in contemporary Britain have a natural and overwhelming motivation for keeping the situation as it is at present. It is follows therefore that it is only when events threaten the status quo, such as the street riots of the early and mid 1980s, that the focus of attention descends on the issue of racism and the role and value of educational approaches within youth work. The way forward appears to lie in youth work finding the space and the commitment to develop and implement approaches that utilize the contradictory position it occupies in British social and cultural life. Society sets youth work the task of containing and socializing young people in its dominant values while offering them activities and facilities that are intended to placate and channel the often unarticulated demands for personal and collective improvement in an unequal and unjust economic and social system. In this scenario youth work can be utilized by progressive practitioners to assist young people to make the cognitive link between their immediate daily condition and the wider social forces that have constructed and perpetuated the situation they find themselves occupying. It is in this context that possibilities can emerge to tackle at a

Whiteness absent

fundamental level racism which is a central feature of both black and white people's lives.

Notes

1. NCWP is an abbreviation for New Commonwealth and Pakistan (the New Commonwealth includes all Commonwealth countries except Australia, Canada and New Zealand).

References

Bhavnani, R. 1986. The struggle for an anti-racist policy in education in Avon. *Critical Social Policy* **16**, 104–8.

Burns, G. 1990. Education, training and black offenders. *Voices* **3**. London: Forum for the Advancement of Training and Education for the Black Unemployed (FATEBU).

Central Statistical Office 1991. *Social Trends 21*. London: HMSO.

Chauhan, V. 1990. *Beyond steel bands 'n' samosas: black young people in the youth service*. Leicester: National Youth Bureau.

Cohen, P. 1988. The perversions of inheritance: studies in the making of multi-racist Britain. In *Multi-racist Britain*, P. Cohen & H. S. Bains (eds). London: Macmillan.

Cole, M. 1989. Monocultural, multicultural and anti-racist education. In *The social contexts of schooling*, M. Cole (ed.). Lewes: Falmer Press.

Craft, A. & G. Klein 1986. *Agenda for multi-cultural teaching*. London: Longman.

CRC 1977. *Seen but not served: black youth and the youth service*. London: Community Relations Commission.

CRE 1980. *Youth in a multi-racial society: the urgent need for new policies*. London: Commission for Racial Equality.

CRE 1983. *Ethnic minority housing staff*. London: Commission for Racial Equality.

CRE 1987. *Overseas doctors: experiences and expectations*. London: Commission for Racial Equality.

Davies, B. 1986. *Threatening youth: towards a national youth policy*. Milton Keynes: Open University Press.

REFERENCES

DES (Department of Education and Science) 1967. *Immigrants and the youth service: report of a Committee for the Youth Service Development Council* (the Hunt Report). London: HMSO.

DES (Department of Education and Science) 1969. Youth and Community Work in the 70s (the Fairbairn–Milson Report). London: HMSO.

Department of Employment 1991. Ethnic origins and the labour market, *Employment Gazette*. February. London: DOE.

Dominelli, L. 1988. *Anti-racist social work: a challenge for white practitioners and educators*. London: Macmillan Education.

Ford, G. 1992. *Fascist Europe: the rise of racism and xenophobia*. London: Pluto Press.

Grinter, R. 1985. Bridging the gulf: the need for an anti-racist multicultural education. *Multi-cultural Teaching* 3(2), 7–10.

Guardian 1993. Brothers in arms fight for the streets. V. Chaudhary and A. Travis. 16–17 October.

Guardian 1994. Fighting talk. G. Younge. 16 March.

Hartley, B. 1971. *The final report of a three year experimental project on coloured teenagers in Great Britain*. Unpublished report, Leicester: National Association of Youth Clubs.

HMSO 1960. The Youth Service in England and Wales (the Albemarle Report) Cmnd. 929. London: HMSO.

HMSO 1982. Experience and Participation. Review Group on the Youth Service in England (the Thompson Report). London: HMSO.

HMSO 1993a. 1991 Census Report for Great Britain. London: HMSO.

HMSO 1993b. 1991 Census Report for Greater London. London: HMSO.

Home Office 1993. Letter to the author from P. Lynch of Home Office. 9 August.

Jeffs, T. & M. Smith 1989. *Using informal education*. Milton Keynes: Open University.

Jeffs, T. & M. Smith 1990. Youth work, youth service and the next few years. *Youth and Policy* 31, 21–9.

Leicester, M. 1986. Multi-cultural Curriculum or Anti-racist Education: Denying the Gulf, cited in M. Cole (1989).

Mayhew, P., D. T. Eliot & L. Dowds 1989. *The 1988 British Crime Survey*. London: HMSO.

Parekh, B. 1986. *The concept of multi-cultural education in multi-cultural education: the interminable debate*. Lewes: Falmer.

Phillips, D. 1987. Searching for a decent home: ethnic minority progress in the post-war housing market. *New Community*, 14. 1/2, 105–47.

Platt, S. 1992. Race wars. *New Statesman and Society*, 5(191),12–13.

Popple, K. 1990. Youth work and race. In *Young people, inequality and youth work*, T. Jeffs and M. Smith (eds). London: Macmillan.

37

Richardson, J. & J. Lambert 1985. *The sociology of race.* Ormskirk: Causeway Press.

Sivanandan, A. 1983. Challenging Racism: Strategies for the Eighties. *Race and Class*, **25**, 1–12.

Sivanandan, A. 1990. *Communities of resistance.* London: Verso.

Smith, M. 1988. *Developing youth work: informal education, mutual aid and popular practice.* Milton Keynes: Open University.

Todd, R. 1991. *Education in a multicultural society.* London: Cassell.

Troyna, B. 1987. A conceptual overview of strategies to combat racial inequality in education: introductory essay. In *Racial inequality in education*, B. Troyna (ed.). London: Tavistock.

Troyna, B. & J. Williams 1986. *Education and the state: the racialisation of education policy.* London: Croom Helm.

Unemployment Unit and Youth Aid 1990. Unemployment Bulletin, **32**, Spring.

Warren, T. 1990. Anti-racist strategies in white working class areas. *Youth and Policy*, **29**, 4–10.

3

Racism in The Netherlands: the challenge for youth policy and youth work

Yvonne Leeman and Sawitri Saharso

Ethnic minorities in The Netherlands

History

The immigrant population of The Netherlands is composed of a wide variety of groups. A distinction can be made between migrants from the former Dutch colonies, migrant labourers, and political refugees and asylum seekers.

During the period of decolonization, many people from the (former) Dutch colonies, that is the Dutch Indies (now Indonesia), Surinam and The Netherlands Antilles, migrated to The Netherlands. Indonesia gained independence in 1949 and in the course of the following ten years approximately 300,000 people moved to The Netherlands. Among them were Moluccans who served as soldiers in the Royal Dutch Indies Army (KNIL) who had fought the Indonesian republicans and were seen as a political problem for both parties. They themselves aspired to a sovereign Moluccan republic. In 1951 they were sent to The Netherlands where upon disembarking they were collectively dismissed from military service. Although the ideal of returning to an independent Moluccan republic is still harboured by many of them, their stay in The Netherlands has turned out to be a permanent one.

The other groups leaving Indonesia, that is the Chinese and Indo-Europeans, came to The Netherlands with the intention of settling permanently. Surinam gained independence in 1975, with the majority of the Surinamese migrants settling in The Netherlands during the late 1960s and in the 1970s. These Surinamese migrants also have diverse ethnic origins: Afro-Caribbean (Creole), Hindustani, Chinese and Javanese. The ethnic composition of the Surinam population is a direct consequence of Dutch colonial policies. First, Africans were "imported" as slaves to work the plantations. The Creoles are their descendants. The Javanese were recruited as contract labour from the Indonesian island of Java in the nineteenth century, followed by Hindustani recruits from the Indian subcontinent. The main motive for their migration was uncertainty of what post-independence would bring them. They were also led by the fear that they would be overruled by the Creoles. The Antilleans mainly came to The Netherlands in the 1950s for further education when the Dutch economy was booming. The majority of Antillean students intended to return to their home country. However, in the 1960s the situation dramatically changed. Computerization and rationalization of the oil industry led to high unemployment and caused working-class people to leave the islands to look for a better future in The Netherlands.

Migrant labour in The Netherlands is not a new phenomenon. Shortly after World War I the first Chinese immigrants settled in The Netherlands. However, the bulk of the people that are today recognized as migrant labourers came after World War II. In the period until 1960 South Europeans, mainly Italians, Spaniards and Yugoslavs, were recruited to work in the coal mines, and the textile and shipbuilding industries. From 1960 the Dutch government started to recruit "guestworkers", as they were called, from Turkey and Morocco, for unskilled work in the old labour-intensive industries. As the term "guestworker" indicates, everybody, the migrant workers included, assumed their stay in The Netherlands would be brief. From 1973, when economic activity decreased, labour recruitment stopped. However, immigration did not stop, with increasing numbers migrating to The Netherlands to rejoin their families.

People fleeing war, violence or persecution in their own country have settled in The Netherlands as invited refugees, in the framework of international quota arrangements made by the UNHCR. Similarly they can arrive on their own initiative. Compared with preceding years the 1980s brought a sharp rise in the second category of people, that is to say people who migrated on their own initiative and appealed for the status of political refugee. The best known among them are probably the Tamils from Sri Lanka and those that have fled the war in former Yugoslavia. In the years between 1986 and 1990 the number of people requesting asylum rose from 5,586 in 1986 to 21,200 in 1990. Not all requesting asylum are granted refugee status. In the period 1990–92 about 10 per cent of requests were granted refugee status and by 1994 a total of 44,000 refugees had been granted asylum.

Immigration and minority policy

As far as immigration is concerned the Dutch government has a policy of "restrictive" admission. "Restrictive" means that a residence permit is only granted on certain grounds. These are: (1) meeting international obligations, (2) cases where fundamental Dutch interests are served, (3) humanitarian cases. The first of these is exemplified by the EU treaty which permits individuals from EU member states the right of residence in another member state for the purpose of employment and other agreed reasons. The contracting of foreign labour to alleviate shortages in the Dutch labour market falls under the second category. The third ground for admission is mainly in cases of family reunion and the granting of asylum to political refugees.

The next basic assumption is that if immigrants are permitted to stay in The Netherlands, their legal and social position should, as much as possible, be equal to that of the indigenous Dutch population. In short, they should become an integral part of Dutch society.

In 1983 the first official government document on immigrants in The Netherlands was published, the so-called "Minority Memorandum". The Memorandum acknowledged that The Netherlands had become a country of immigration, and immigrants were likely to stay in the country. The Memorandum not only stated that the immigrants had come for permanent settlement, but also recognized their current marginal social and economic position. Therefore a minority policy was launched that was directed at (1) addressing their deprivation, (2) promoting their social integration, and (3) combating racism and discrimination. In practice the minority policy has become oriented towards the second target, social integration, with "labour" as the main instrument through which the integration is to be achieved.

The six most important target groups of the minority policy are: Surinamese, Turks, Moroccans, Moluccans, Antilleans, and South Europeans. In the rest of this overview we will concentrate on these six groups which consist in all of some 950,000 people. It is now over 10 years since the minority policy came into operation. What has happened to the people it was concerned with, and how did they fare during those years? These questions are addressed in a study by Veenman (1994) and the following is mainly based on his work.

Demography

At the time of writing, of a total Netherlands population of 15 million approximately 1.5 million people are from an immigrant background forming some 10 per cent of the population. Not all migrants are subject to the national minority policy that is in particular directed at immigrant groups with a low socio-economic status. In 1992 the Surinamese were the largest group with 263,000 members with an average length of residence in The

Netherlands of almost 14 years. The second largest group were the Turks with 241,000 members and an average length of residence of 12 years. The third group, the Moroccans, had 96,000 members and the same length of residence as the Turks. The Antillean group consisted of 91,000 people with an average length of residence of 9.5 years, and the Moluccan group was estimated to consist of 37,500 people with an average length of residence of 30 years.

All the groups mentioned have in the last ten years increased in number. This is largely due to an increase in the birth rate and continuing immigration, neither of which was expected by policy makers. The Dutch government, which has adopted a policy of restrictive admission towards immigrants, has long ceased recruiting migrant workers and since family reunion is more or less completed, it was expected that the immigration would decrease. In practice this has not happened, primarily because many young people marry a partner from their country of origin. For example, the growth of the Turkish group in 1990 is explained by about two thirds from immigration and one third by natural growth.

The migrant groups are very unevenly distributed over The Netherlands and are particularly concentrated in the four large cities of Amsterdam, Rotterdam, The Hague and Utrecht where they are predominantly housed in low status neighbourhoods. In 1994, in the city of Amsterdam, the percentage of youngsters between the ages of 0 and 20 belonging to ethnic minorities was 45 per cent, and in Rotterdam 35 per cent.

The socio-economic position

Ethnic minorities in The Netherlands are associated with poverty and low socio-economic status. This situation holds for most, but not all, people who have migrated to The Netherlands. The main exceptions are the Indo-Europeans, who in general have prospered in Dutch society, and the South Europeans, who have in the past decade proved to be an upwardly mobile group. The Indo-Europeans have therefore never been targeted by the Dutch minority policy and at the time of writing it is questionable whether it is appropriate that the South Europeans should continue to be considered within this policy.

How then did 950,000 people who form the target groups for the minority policy fare during the last decade? Compared with their position ten years ago, their situation has improved, but compared with the indigenous population it has worsened. The achievement level in education of immigrant youth, for instance, is higher than that of their parents but still lower than that of their indigenous peers.

The unemployment figures for the various migrant groups decreased in the second half of the 1980s, but are still very high, certainly when compared with the unemployment rate of the Dutch. The percentage unemployment figures for 1990–91 illustrate the point: Turks 31 per cent, Moroccans 36 per cent, Surinamese 26 per cent, Antilleans 31 per cent, Moluccans 17 per cent, compared to the Dutch at 7 per cent. Migrants not only have higher unemployment rates, they are also more likely to be long-term unemployed.

When we look at job levels, promotional opportunities and labour quality the following picture arises. Of the four largest immigrant groups, the Turks and Moroccans work in the most menial jobs, while the Surinamese and Antilleans occupy a middle position. The labour position of immigrant groups is also characterized by a very uneven spread over occupational groups and branches of industry. Immigrant men and women are over-represented in industrial occupations and under-represented in commercial occupations, management positions, and particularly in academic jobs.

The income of migrant groups is strongly related to their labour position. First, the number of people that are dependent on social security is much higher among migrants than among Dutch people. Second, the monthly income of those migrants who obtain their income through paid work is, on average,

Dfl. 350 to Dfl. 450 less than that of the indigenous Dutch. Again, the income of Turks, Surinamese and Moroccans is the worst of all categories being heavily over-represented in the lowest labour income groups with a net income of less than Dfl. 1,500 per month.

The poor labour position of the above-mentioned migrant groups is explained by several factors with Veenman (1994) pointing to a succession of economic recessions, a radical and far-reaching and, for migrants, unfavourable economic restructuring which has led to a drastic reduction in unskilled and manual jobs, and a reluctance by many employers to hire migrants.

As far as housing conditions are concerned we have already mentioned the concentration of migrants in certain areas in large cities. The houses in such areas are usually old, cramped and situated in the inner cities. When more than 50 per cent of an area is occupied by migrants we consider this an area of concentration. Almost 75 per cent of the Turks and Moroccans are living in such areas, compared to half of the Surinamese and Antillean population and 40 per cent of the indigenous Dutch. For several years after their arrival Moluccans were accommodated in special housing projects in certain assigned areas. At present 80 per cent of Moluccans are still living in these areas, and half of them continue to reside in the same housing projects to which they were originally allocated. Since the 1970s many have moved to the big cities, where now some 20 per cent are housed in the areas of concentration. It is not just that people from a migrant background are concentrated in such areas. Similarly, as low income earners they are likely to suffer from unemployment, live in low-quality housing conditions, and their children are likely to have poor school results. Ghettoization is therefore now considered to be a serious problem by policy makers.

Racism and anti-racism in The Netherlands

Traditionally The Netherlands has the reputation of being an open democratic society in which there is no room for racism. This image of "Dutch tolerance" has been damaged in the last two decades by several phenomena.

Since the 1980s a number of studies of young people have demonstrated that many of them are prejudiced and a large number of them harbour hostile feelings against blacks and migrants. A survey carried out in the early 1980s among 4,800 students in the highest grades of 15 secondary schools indicated that 27 per cent of respondents had a negative attitude towards ethnic minorities and 8 per cent held extreme right-wing views (Hagendoorn & Janssen 1983). This survey was replicated among students in the lowest level of secondary schools and showed that 46 per cent of them scored above average on the ethnocentrism scale with a hard core of 14 per cent harbouring extreme intolerant feelings against migrants (Raaijmakers 1986). The national survey among pupils in secondary education (Scholierenonderzoek 1992) indicated that 32 per cent of boys and 24 per cent of girls considered "the presence of other cultures in The Netherlands" to be an important social problem, as important as AIDS, unemployment and drugs. Finally, Kleinpenning (1993) found that 44.8 per cent of the young people in his national survey agreed with one or more racist pronouncements. These studies have made use of sociometric questionnaires and give no insight into possible ambivalencies in the attitude and opinions of young people and can therefore only be considered to be a rough guide to the attitudes of Dutch youth. Unfortunately, qualitative studies which might offer more helpful insights are scarce.

In 1977 the first recorded fatality of racist violence was that of a Turkish man who was drowned after being thrown into a canal. A well-known incident was the murder, in August 1983, of the 15-year-old Antillean boy, Kerwin Duinmeyer, by a 16-year-old skinhead. Violent acts against migrants include intimidation, threats, the "blackening" of victims, arson, fights (some of which end in death), maltreatment, shootings and bomb attacks.

As an indication of the kind of racist violence and the extent to which it occurs, we present the following racist incidents documented by van Donselaar (1993) for the year 1992. A series of attacks on mosques started with an attack with fire bombs on a mosque in the city of Amersfoort, followed shortly after by attacks on seven other mosques. Then followed a series of violent acts in the city of The Hague. In a period of four months there were four fire-bomb attacks, three cases of arson, three (false) bomb scares, four cases of building demolition and several cases of maltreatment. The worst case concerned the violent beating up and kicking of a Haitian man by a group of five young skinheads, one of whom was active in a racist party.

In 1971 racism was for the first time politically expressed through the founding of the Dutch Peoples' Union (Nederlandse Volks Unie, NVU). This single issue political party had as its political mission, "Foreigners out!", and was widely known for its scathing agitation against the presence of migrants in The Netherlands. In 1980 the NVU was joined by the Centre Party (Centrumpartij, CP), which differed in strategy from the NVU, although not in its goals. In the elections of 1982, its leader, Janmaat, gained a seat in Parliament. While the NVU no longer exists the CP rose again, having survived several internal conflicts in 1984, and has since then been a more or less permanent factor in politics. It succeeded, for instance, in winning 2.5 per cent of votes in the elections for Parliament held in May 1994. This means they are represented by three seats in Parliament.

The NVU and CP had (and the CP still has) their youth organizations, respectively the National Youth Front (National Jeugd Front) and the Young Beggars (Jonge Geuzen). Next to be mentioned are the The Netherlands Youth Front (Jongeren Front Nederland, JFN), which was disbanded in 1990, the Viking Youth (Viking Jeugd), and the Action Front National Socialists (Actiefront Nationaal Socialisten, ANS). These organizations are loosely supported by many militant youth (mainly skinheads) but it is not clear to what organization, if any, they belong.

Racism and racist discrimination is forbidden by law in The Netherlands and people and organizations that break the law can be prosecuted and punished. Both the national government and local councils have developed anti-racist policies. The Amsterdam council, for instance, has developed an anti-racist policy which is coordinated by the (municipal) bureau strategic minority policy. The target groups are municipal organizations and citizens, institutions, companies and industries. Among the measures taken are positive action, contract compliance, an anti-discrimination code; a financed anti-discrimination bureau to which people can turn with their complaints, and an annual media reward for journalists. Municipal anti-racist demonstrations are also financed, such as the annual memorial commemorating the death of Kerwin Duinmeyer.

There are four national organizations engaged in fighting racism. These are the Workshop for Law & Race Discrimination founded in 1983, the National Office Combating Racism, also founded in 1983, the Anne Frank Foundation, founded in 1957, and the Anti-Discrimination Consultancy, founded in 1987. Although complaints about racism and discrimination should, in order to be prosecuted, ultimately be made to the police, the step to the police is for many too great. Therefore in several cities anti-discrimination bureaux or complaints centres have been established, run by volunteers and financed by local governments.

Racism: youth policy and youth work

Youth policy

"The development of the multicultural society is accompanied by problems like racism", is a statement made in the policy paper on intersectorial youth policy entitled "Youth deserves the future" (Ministry of Welfare, Health and Culture, 1993: 57). In order to strengthen the work of state and local authorities, institutions, organizations and individuals in their fight against racism, an activity programme for young people has been designed. This programme, which is part of the general ethnic minorities policy, contains a range of measures that have anti-racism as a common theme. If we were to characterize with keywords the different measures taken in regard to and on behalf of youth, these would be "ban racism", "prevention" and "participation". "Participation" corresponds to one of the main targets of the general ethnic minorities policy. It is assumed that a high rate of participation by ethnic minorities at all levels of society provides the best impetus for tolerance. Closely connected with participation is the aim of preventing the social marginalization of young people in general and of ethnic youth in particular. In the following discussion on the initiatives taken we will concentrate on the range of activities which is directly aimed at influencing the attitudes and beliefs of young people in the direction of anti-racism and tolerance.

Different ministries play a part in youth policy. The central department in the development of youth policy is the Ministry of Health, Welfare and Sport (VWS), but measures on behalf of migrant youth often fall under the minority policy that is coordinated by the Ministry of Home Affairs (BiZa). The third partner is the Ministry of Education, Culture and Science (OCW). In trying to avoid a fragmented national and local policy there is a strong emphasis on achieving coherence and mutual understanding between different departments. Since the 1980s there has been a move to decentralize welfare and youth policy in The Netherlands. Instead of merely carrying out national policy, local authorities have more freedom in designing and initiating a coherent local policy. Decentralization offers the possibility of a policy to correspond with local needs and problems. It also facilitates the direct participation of members of target groups in the planning of policy and initiatives. In describing youth policy in The Netherlands one is aware of a very complex picture. There scarcely exists any specific youth policy. It is predominantly integrated in policies on welfare, education and employment. Therefore initiatives on youth and anti-racism are financed by, and part of, the policy of different national departments or of local authorities.

The banning of racism, which is one of the targets of the ethnic minorities policy, within the national youth policy, is mainly translated into the distribution of information. There are many ways to reach young people with a message of anti-racism and tolerance. On a local level there is an emphasis on youth work to reach young people. National initiatives use schools or youth organizations as intermediaries or try to reach young people directly through computer games, exhibitions or concerts. Depending on the method chosen, one can expect to more or less reach young people. The project "Pop Against Racism" is an example of a direct approach which has proved to be successful. Established in Amsterdam in 1993, "Pop Against Racism" organizes every year a massive free pop festival called "Racism Beat It" which is attended by thousands of young people from all over The Netherlands. Besides listening to music young people can also visit an information market where anti-racist organizations sell their T-shirts, badges and posters. At the festival in September 1994 a survey undertaken among visitors indicated that most were well educated. The main reason given by respondents for visiting the festival was the theme of anti-racism, then for the music and the pleasant atmosphere. 86 per cent of the visitors believed the festival contributed towards the advancement of tolerance.

These results demonstrate that "Pop Against Racism" is successful in reaching a large number of young people, in particular those interested in anti-racism. In order to reach youngsters who have an indifferent attitude towards anti-racism, or to reach young right-wing extremists, one has to choose a different tack.

Youth work

Youth work is situated at the municipal and community level and is generally undertaken by private welfare organizations. It is possible to distinguish between support-oriented and socio-cultural youth work. For our discussion we have concentrated on socio-cultural youth work. Over the years community-oriented youth work has focused on youth at risk, offering predominantly indigenous Dutch young people a place of their own to meet each other. For those young people participating it is something like a "second home". The contacts between staff and young people are very informal with little emphasis on the pedagogical role of the workers. In general immigrant youth do not participate in community-oriented youth work which tends to be run by Dutch adults for Dutch young people.

Youth work also takes place in "open" youth centres which serve the whole city and are directly financed by the municipality. These centres usually function as a place for pop music and theatre. Some centres are organized by and for immigrant young people, which means there are few opportunities for them to mix with Dutch youth.

In situations where youth workers are confronted with problems between youth of different ethnic origin, their response has been to prevent difficulties. Separating groups from each other by developing different activities at varying hours or places is the common strategy used in community-oriented youth work (NIZW 1993). In this type of youth work there is little experience with programmes that concentrate on anti-racism and on the development of respect and tolerance for ethnic diversity (NIZW 1993). Youth workers confronted with racist views and extreme right-wing youth have found an answer by developing an anti-discrimination code combined with presenting clear values condemning racism. The commemoration in 1995 of the 50th anniversary of the end of the Second World War provided an opportunity to prioritize the subject of tolerance. At the same time there is, after neglect of more than a decade, a tendency to re-examine the pedagogical mission of this type of youth work. Due to these developments there is a growing interest in methods that influence young people, in particular those who express racist or intolerant views. Although youth workers are in need of assistance in this area only meagre resources are available. Those few initiatives that are undertaken are poorly documented and evaluated. One of the exceptions is the local initiative "Wereldkinderen" (Children of the World) which we will now discuss in more detail.

The project "Children of the World" is an initiative by youth workers based at two different youth centres, one for the Dutch and one for Morrocan youth living in Maastricht. The main purpose of the project is to bring Dutch youngsters in contact with their peers from immigrant backgrounds who are living in the same neighbourhood. In turn the project offers Moroccan youth the opportunity to meet Dutch young people. The project has focused on so-called "problematic" youth, that is those living in poor circumstances, having poor school results, engaged in the drugs scene, etc. "Children of the World" is a purposeful attempt to make contacts between young people of different ethnic background and indigenous Dutch youth. The emphasis is on action rather than talking, meeting each other for sporting events, visiting other places or exhibitions, or making a trip of several days together. The project, which lasted one year, had a core group of 18 boys, half of them Dutch and half of them Moroccan, all between 16 and 25 years old. About fifty youngsters, boys and some girls, participated in the activities which were planned and organized by a small group of five boys who represented both youth centres. For these five boys, who were key figures in mobilizing their friends to join in, it was an exercise in taking responsibility and in developing different skills, such as organizing and planning. That the project met its aims is evidenced by Abdrahim, a boy of Moroccan descent.

I joined the activity because Driss asked me to. I don't really know the Dutch. I mainly see them, but I never genuinely talk with them. They seem so closed to me and overbearing. Or they think that you are a dealer. But all I want is simply to live unnoticed, to work and to earn money and to be happy with my family. I was very happy when I noticed that the other boys were interested in me. We talk about praying, school in Morocco and I learned something about their life at home. They also have strict fathers and mothers. I have to try to learn better Dutch, as I want to stay in touch with those boys.

As they became acquainted they started to talk and exchange experiences with each other and became a group themselves. This was intensified by presenting themselves as a group to the outside world. For example they gave an interview to the local newspaper and pictures taken of the activities were exhibited in both centres.

Among the activities were visits to a migrant information centre, an exhibition on discrimination in The Netherlands, the celebration of the Islamic Slaughter Feast, and a visit to a former concentration camp for Jews. The visit to the concentration camp deeply impressed the boys. Huub, a Dutch boy, said after the visit,

> You watch exciting, rough films about the war and it looks like a survival in the Ardennes. Then you come here and you are in a cold sweat. Something like this, no, it is impossible! To destroy people because they think in a different way or have a different appearance, it is just an impossible thing to do to hurl them away like rubbish. I can't understand that there is over there again a crowd, which yell the same things. Now it is against Moroccans and refugees. You should get them over here to make them see this. That will immediately cure them of that insanity.

Another Dutch boy, Tommy, said after the visit,

When you have seen this with brown, black, red or blue eyes, there is only one thing left to say: "We have to see to it that those fucking idiots never seize power again." It is not normal to destroy people in a way worse than pigs and chickens, only because they appear different.

Although the project does not have an explicit anti-racist message and moral, as the utterances of Huub and Tommy show, the message is easily conveyed through the activities. The project is not focused on a negative approach like "you should not discriminate", but on a positive approach which is aimed at respect and tolerance developed through collective activities. This approach links up well with current methods in youth work.

Characteristic of community-oriented and open youth work is the voluntary participation of young people. With the theme of learning by doing, informal learning is very popular. The strong accent on active participation of youngsters in the organization and creation of activities makes the "Children of the World" initiative easily transferable to others.

The main principles of "Children of the World" are reflected in the present activities within the framework of the "Youth Projects for Friendship and Tolerance" which is part of the "Colourful Euregion" initiative. In these projects, youngsters from Belgium, Germany and The Netherlands, who live in the land between the rivers Rhine and Maas, and who represent various ethnic groups, have the opportunity to meet each other and work together on common activities in the areas of art, music and sport. Here again there is a positive approach to a multi-ethnic society and a strong emphasis on active participation and working together with young people from different backgrounds. At the time of writing, this approach is considered by youth workers as the most promising in creating and sustaining tolerance.

The school as an intermediary

Many locally and nationally funded initiatives in the domain of youth and the multi-ethnic society use schools as an intermediary to influence young people. Since attending school is compulsory, it is through the schools that organizations hope to reach the average boy or girl. Schools, however, have a generally limited interest in subject matters related to the multi-ethnic society. Nevertheless many organizations have developed education packs as a supplement to the standard curriculum. An important initiative in this area are the yearly editions of the *Anne Frankkrant* published by the Anne Frank Foundation. These are full-colour magazines for young people from 10 to 14 years and for youngsters above the age of 14. The distribution is once a year through primary and secondary schools. The magazine contains subjects such as information about Anne Frank, the Second World War and discussions on anti-Semitism, racism and discrimination. Financial assistance from local municipalities has enabled the magazines to reach a wide readership.

Another interesting initiative that supplements the school curriculum is "Face to Face", a media project that brings together different countries and cultures. The target audience is young people in secondary schools, with special attention paid to those young people from ethnic minority groups who want to find their way around the media world. The pupils of a school class communicate with the pupils of a school in another country using video letters, written letters and E-mail. They are given an opportunity to share and discuss their personal experiences while being introduced to the workings of the media business. A "Face to Face" project covers the duration of a school year, during which time each participating class sends two video letters. An exchange of video letters opens up a world of two-way communication with participants receiving personal messages from pupils and teachers in another country. They can see each other's faces and voices, and each other's living conditions and working environment. They are communicating "Face to Face". The "Face to

Face" project started in 1990 with two ethnically mixed secondary school classes in Amsterdam and New York. By 1994 some
100 classes world wide were communicating with video letters.
"Face to Face" is a part of an equal opportunities project of
the Foreigners Media-network Foundation, which offers young
people from ethnic minority groups a taste of the media world
including script writing, operating a camera, editing and so
forth. One of the project's main objectives is to encourage immigrant young people to make a career in the media. Young people
entering the media world is a goal for the project as a way of fur-
thering equal opportunities. At the same time Dutch youngsters
become acquainted with people from ethnic minorities working
within radio, television and newspapers. It is hoped that this will
aid the development of respect and tolerance. The project as a
whole is a good example of the practice of the Dutch policy on
ethnic minorities, with its strong emphasis on the participation of
minority groups as a means to developing respect and tolerance.

"School without Racism" is an initiative that makes use of
the school in a different way. This project is not focused on the
curriculum but on the school as a community. "School without
Racism" is an international movement which was launched in
Belgium and The Netherlands. In The Netherlands the local
foundation for the welfare of foreigners started in spring 1994
with campaigns to encourage school pupils to take initiatives to
reject racism and promote tolerance. The pupils are asked to
prove, on the basis of a petition, that at least 70 per cent of the
school population, pupils and teachers, want to have a "School
without Racism". This title, which is displayed on a specially
made plaque, also implies obligations. When a school has declared itself as a "School without Racism" it has to take action
against any utterance of racism within the school and has to provide intercultural education and promote a climate of tolerance
for ethnic diversity. It is important that the initiative is in the
hands of the pupils themselves and by collecting support for the
petition they are automatically obliged to discuss racism with
their fellow pupils and with teachers. These discussions can

strengthen the support for anti-racism in a more effective way than merely introducing an anti-discrimination code in schools, which can easily remain words and not be translated into action. The initiative has proved quite successful and after less than a year of campaigning 15 schools have already gained a plaque. Pupils who represent over a hundred different schools (out of a total of a thousand secondary schools in The Netherlands) are now busy collecting signatures.

In summary, we have noted that The Netherlands offers a complex picture of national and local initiatives on young people, anti-racism and tolerance. The initiatives are poorly co-ordinated at the national level, being part of the policy of different ministries as well as a component of policy at a decentralized level. The initiatives are dependent on local city authorities who co-ordinate them, with different degrees of energy and success. Youth work does not automatically extend to the average young person, and organizations that want to reach them with a message of non-discrimination and tolerance often opt for the school as an intermediary.

In general there is a lack of knowledge and experience about methods that interest and influence young people in the area of anti-racism and tolerance. We do know, however, that some local youth-work initiatives are proving to be successful. Their methodology is characterized by both its positive message of a multiethnic society and its strong emphasis on active participation and working together with young people from different backgrounds.

Research

Most of the research in the area of youth, youth policy and youth work is financed by national authorities which influence the objectives and research methods used. Research which has youth as its main focus tends to neglect ethnic differences and young people's perspective on a multi-ethnic society. An example is the study "Being young and growing up in The Netherlands" (van der Linden & Dijkman 1989) which provides a view of the lives of 500 adolescents. The research was financed in order to serve as a basis for the development of future youth policy. The outcome is a policy that does not differentiate along ethnic lines and pays little attention to The Netherlands being a multi-ethnic society.

This is different from the general policy on ethnic minorities which pays special attention to immigrant youth. The research undertaken in this setting is mainly concerned with the goals of participation and the integration of immigrant young people. Consequently most of the research in this field can be characterized as research aimed at monitoring the position of ethnic youth and comparing it with the position of Dutch young people (Veenman 1994; Junger 1990). As a consequence immigrant youngsters are predominantly viewed as representatives of their ethnic group by virtue of being part of "another culture". The bulk of this type of research focuses on only one category of ethnic youth: youth at risk. Most of the studies are on Moroccan and Surinamese boys who are almost, or are already, marginalized, or girls who run away from home or who refuse to attend school (Sansone 1984, 1990; Werdmölder 1986, 1990; Kaufman & Verbeck 1986). The result of this type of research is the construction of ethnic youth as "problematic youth" and a category which is in all respects "different" from their Dutch contemporaries. While some research has been undertaken in the field of prejudice, racism and the inter-ethnic community, most results in superficial insights because the main research method is survey work rather than interviews with the young people. A further problem of this research has been the focus upon the individual "racist".

The trend in Dutch research is therefore to ignore immigrant young people, or to present them as very different from Dutch youngsters who are viewed as individuals with prejudices against people from other backgrounds. The research is rarely based upon searching interviews with young people themselves and does not take into consideration any situational analysis of racism or the nature of inter-ethnic relationships. In our recent work

(Leeman & Saharso 1989; Saharso 1992; Leeman 1994) we therefore concentrate on detailed interviews with immigrant and Dutch young people. We were interested in the meaning they gave to their experiences of living in a mixed ethnic community. As we did not want to consider the youngsters in advance as representatives of two mutually excluded groups of immigrant and Dutch young people, we conceptualized ethnic identity as a social identity that is integrated in, but also distinct from, a person's individual sense of identity. In our view, personal and social identity do not fully coincide and therefore young people can choose between several identity options. Interviewing contemporary youth produced an interesting picture of the differences and similarities between young people in their relationship to a mixed ethnic community. In Leeman and Saharso (1989, 1991) we show the different ways that racism is dealt with by Moluccan, Surinamese and Moroccan young people. We relate these differences to their differing historical relationship with The Netherlands and to their divergent traditions. Saharso (1992) provides an account of the life stories of 42 young people from various ethnic minority groups including youngsters from Surinam, Turkey, Morocco, Pakistan, Spain, the Antilles and adolescents of Indo-European origin. Paying particular attention to ethnic identity, friendship and discrimination, Saharso demonstrates the different ways in which ethnicity may acquire meaning in a person's life. It was found that how youngsters relate to their ethnicity depends on their personality, their personal circumstances and their group's history. For some, their ethnic identity has an important role in counterbalancing their experiences of discrimination and marginalization and they are drawn to cultivate their ethnic identity. Children of immigrant contract workers are sharply aware of the fact that their parents moved to The Netherlands to find a better life. They have been strongly motivated to succeed in their country of adoption only to find that their ethnicity is not valued in society. They usually experience their ethnicity as a self-evident and, at the same time, unimportant part of their personality.

Notwithstanding these mutual differences, the immigrant youngsters interviewed share similarities. Because of their experienced discrimination most of them feel that they are forced into, and subjectively identify with, the category of "foreigners". So, although emotionally they may identify with a specific ethnic group, they also feel they are foreigners in The Netherlands. This developing shared identity as foreigners does not necessarily exclude Dutch young people. Leeman (1994) portrays Dutch youth as classmates of the secondary school youngsters portrayed by Saharso. She sketches a diverse picture of Dutch youngsters in their relationship with ethnic young people. When questioned about ethnic differences the Dutch youngsters demonstrated some interesting local differences. For example, for young people attending schools in the ethnically heterogeneous environment of the large Dutch cities of Amsterdam and The Hague the general view of immigrant youngsters was that they were "just like everyone else": after all they had grown up together. Young Dutch people from smaller, less ethnically heterogenous towns like Dordrecht and Zaandam reported a greater social distance between themselves and immigrant youngsters.

Leeman found that young people living in big cities more frequently had an ethnically mixed circle of friends than youngsters living in smaller towns. Growing up together in the same neighbourhood was found to be more influential in young people's development than their ethnic differences. Within this pattern of local differences it is not enough only to take the ethnic composition of the town or of the neighbourhood into account. Other features of the local situation that need to be considered are the local mutual ideological representation and the balance of power between immigrant and Dutch young people (see also Hewitt 1986). In Amsterdam for instance, many of the youngsters whom we interviewed, both immigrant and Dutch, were members of groups that hung about on street corners and in city squares. Most of these groups were made up of immigrant young people, and the Dutch young people who were part of the group were considered to be "part of us foreigners". Dutch youngsters who

CONCLUSION

associate with immigrant young people in this way could be considered to be anti-racist, but it is also a matter of style and being seen to be "cool".

A situational analysis of inter-ethnic relationships combined with an insight into the meaning given to these by young people of different origins provides an indication of the possibilities of youth work that challenges racism. What is required now in The Netherlands is the development of methods that can be used in youth work to account for the different ways in which youngsters experience racism. The conditions for these methods, however, are unfavourable, and the developmental and evaluation research is scarce, hampering the dissemination of the experience and knowledge gained so far.

Conclusion

We have seen that the immigrant population of The Netherlands is composed of a wide variety of groups that are concentrated in the country's four largest cities. They share a low socio-economic status which is in part caused by racism.

The image of "Dutch tolerance" no longer represents reality in The Netherlands today. Racist political parties have won their way into parliament, racist incidents are part of everyday life, and surveys among Dutch young people indicate that a substantial number of them are prejudiced and exhibit hostile feelings against immigrants.

Since the 1980s the Dutch government has developed a minority policy, aimed at improving the social position of immigrant groups. Although in practice the policy is focused at the integration of ethnic minorities, it is also aimed at combating racism. It is believed that intensifying the participation of ethnic minorities at all levels of society is the best way of increasing tolerance. Among the measures taken by national and local authorities are positive action and the establishment of anti-discrimination codes. Several national organizations that are in receipt of state finance are engaged in fighting racism.

The Netherlands offers a complex picture of national and local initiatives on youth, anti-racism and tolerance. The national youth policy of challenging racism has been translated into the distribution of information. We mentioned the "Pop against Racism" project that is directed both at socializing young people from different ethnic backgrounds and at the distribution of information.

Youth work is located at the municipal level and we have seen that community-orientated youth work focuses mainly on Dutch young people. In addition there exist open youth centres. Some of these are organized by and for immigrant youth. This means that Dutch and immigrant young people are not likely to meet in youth settings. Youth workers who are confronted by youngsters with intolerant feelings have expressed the need for methods to deal with these attitudes but there are few initiatives in this field and these are poorly documented. We have discussed the project "Children of the World" which is aimed at bringing Dutch young people with racist views into contact with immigrant youngsters, in particular Moroccans, living in the same neighbourhood. The project's approach has been to focus on the development of mutual respect and tolerance through collective activities and it has been shown that the anti-racist message was more easily, and probably better, conveyed through such activities than by any explicit moral lesson.

Many initiatives use the school to influence young people. Every year the *Anne Frankkrant*, a magazine for young people between the ages of 10 and 14 years, is produced and distributed to schools. We noted the "Face to Face" media project that through video letters, written letters and E-mail brings together youngsters from different countries and cultures.

We have also discussed research into the experiences of youngsters and their attitude towards a mixed ethnic community. The results indicate the need to avoid forcing young people to perceive the world in terms of ethnic categories. By avoiding these categories we find that we can discover the actual views and experiences of contemporary youth. Such a research approach is more in line with the aim of developing a dynamic multi-ethnic society in which ethnic boundaries are transcended rather than built.

The challenge now for youth work in The Netherlands is to develop methods that bring together young people from different ethnic backgrounds and to offer them an anti-racist programme. In this respect some local initiatives look very promising. In such projects there is a strong emphasis on the active involvement and working together of young people from different ethnic backgrounds. Another important aspect of those projects is that they provide individuals with responsibilities, which we think is the key to a future of tolerance.

Notes

1. The complete list of the target groups of the minority policy consists of: Surinamese and Antillians; Moluccans; migrant workers and their families from recruitment countries; gypsies; refugees; and the Dutch group of caravan dwellers.

References and further reading

Donselaar, J. van 1993. Racistisch geweld en extreem-recht, *Migrantenstudies*, 3, 2–15.
Gemeente Amsterdam 1993. *Beleidsnota stedelijk jongerenwerk*, gemeenteblad, bijlage L.
Hagendoorn L. & J. Janssen 1983. *Rechts-omkeer: rechts-extreme opvattingen bij Leerlingen van middelbare scholen*. Baarn: Ambo.
Hewitt, R. 1986. *White talk, black talk. Inter-racial friendship and communication amongst adolescents*. Cambridge: Cambridge University Press.
Jaarboek Minderheden 1995. Bohn Stafleu Van Loghum: Houten/ Zaventem.

Junger, M. 1990. *Delinquency and ethnicity. An investigation on social factors relating to delinquency among Moroccan, Turkish, Surinamese and Dutch boys*. Derenter: Kluwer Law and Taxation.

Kaufman, P. & H. Verbeck 1986. *Marokkaan en verslaafd*. Utrecht.

Kleinpenning, G. 1993. *Structure and content of racist beliefs*. Utrecht: ISOR.

Leeman, Y. 1994. *Samen jong. Nederlandse jongeren en lessen over interetnisch samenleven en discriminatie*. Utrecht: Van Arkel.

Leeman, Y. & S. Saharso 1989. *Je kunt er niet omheen. Hoe Marokkaanse, Molukse en Surinaamse jongeren reageren op discriminatie*, Amsterdam/Lisse: Swets & Zeitlinger.

Leeman, Y. & S. Saharso 1991. Coping with discrimination. *European Journal of Intercultural Studies*, Spring 1(3), 5–17.

Linden, F. Th. van der & Dijkman 1989. *Jong zijn en volwassen worden in Nederland*. Nijmegen: Hoogveld Instituut.

Ministry of Welfare, Health and Culture 1993. *Jeugd verdient de toekomst*. Rijswijk: Ministry of Welfare, Health and Culture.

NIZW, 1993, *Jeugdwerk rond 4 en 5 mei*, Utrecht: NIZW.

Raaijmakers, Q. 1986. Verrechtsing en politieke intolerantie bij middelbare scholieren. In *Beelden van jeugd*, M. Matthijssen (ed.). Groningen: Wolters-Noordhoff.

Saharso, S. 1989. Ethnic identity and the Paradox of Equality. In *Ethnic minorities: social pychological perspectives*, J. P. Oudenhoven & T. M. Willemsen (eds). Amsterdam/Lisse: Swets & Zeitlinger.

Saharso, S. 1992. *Jan en alleman. Etnische jeugd over etnische identiteit, discriminatie en vriendschap*. Utrecht: Van Arkel.

Sansone, L. 1984. *... and leisure time is mine. The Creole youth of Amsterdam in social welfare, vocational education and leisure time*. Amsterdam: Afdeling Bestuursin formatë.

Sansone, L. 1990. *Lasi boto. De boot gemist. Over Surinaamse jongeren, werk en werkloosheid*. Amersfoort/Leuven: Acco.

Scholierenonderzoek 1992. Nibud, Zeitlinger Den Haags.

Trajekt, 1993. *Project Wereldjongeren*, Maastricht: Trajekt.

Veenman, J. 1994. *Participatie in perspectief. Ontwikkelingen in de sociaaleconomische positie van zes allochtone groepen in Nederland*. Bohn Stafleu van Loghum, Houten/Zaventem.

Vries, M. de 1987. *Ogen in je rug. Turkse meisjes en jonge vrouwen in Nederland*. Alphen a/d Rijn: Samson.

Werdmölder, H. 1986. *Van vriendenkring tot randgroep. Marokkaanse jongeren in een oude stadswijk*. Houten: Gouda Quint.

Werdmölder, H. 1990. *Een generatie op drift. De geschiedenis van een Marokkaanse randgroep*. Arnhem.

4

Emigration to immigration: young people in a changing Spain

Pablo Angel Meira Cartea and
José Antonio Caride Gómez

Introduction: migration processes and social reality

In the last few decades Spain has undergone a great deal of political, economic and social reform. These reforms are the result of both changes within Spain and transformations that have occurred in the geo-political and economic world order. Changes have also taken place in the Spanish demographic structure in relation to its birth and death rates and in migration processes. These have all generated new challenges and new social problems.

In the mid 1970s Spain began its delicate transition from dictatorship to democracy, with official approval of the present Constitution given on 6 December 1978. Spain is now defined as a "Constitutional Social Democratic State" in which the fundamental values are liberty, justice and equality. Political pluralism is adhered to within a system of parliamentary democracy. Different levels of territorial and political autonomy have been acknowledged, leading to regional and national groups playing a part in the country's future. On a socio-economic level all productive sectors have assisted the country to move from one of peripheral influence to one that is fully engaged in international activities, particularly in world trade, in commerce and capital, as

65

well as involvement in modernization processes and technological innovation.

Although Spain has moved from an agricultural to a modern advanced society and has established strong industrial and service sectors, there remain distinct regional inequalities in the distribution and provision of the means of production, and in levels of income and the quality of life for citizens. The incorporation of Spain into the European Community on 1 January 1986 further assisted its economic development. As noted by Tamames (1994) during the period 1986 to 1990 the Spanish economy experienced a significant expansion with a yearly growth rate of 5 per cent. From 1994 to the time of writing there has been a change with a recession-hit economy. For example, the unemployment rate in 1995 has been registered at 22 per cent of the economically active population with more than 3 million people seeking employment, the majority of whom are young people looking for their first job.

The search for solutions to the socio-economical problems has led to an important debate within Spanish society. The government have committed themselves to measures that have encouraged incentives and the flexibility of labour, and which have brought with them opposition from the trade unions. During the mid 1990s government initiatives had the effect of increasing the number of jobs available and reducing unemployment rates, while liberalizing contract conditions and introducing insecurity in the labour market.

Emigration: Spain as a country of origin

The changes in the Spanish economy since the 1960s have been accompanied by identifiable migratory patterns. One that took place mainly between 1960 and 1970 was the movement of people from regions that had few opportunities for economic growth to those regions and cities where there was increased scope for work, improved living conditions and an increased quality of life. In general the movements have meant people leaving small villages, leading to the depopulation of large areas of rural Spain. At the same time urban areas developed in an excessive and unplanned manner. The problems associated with this migration have been linked to the scarcity of housing, marginalization, and the inability of numbers of people to satisfactorily adapt to their new place of settlement.

Traditionally, Spain has been a country of emigration. From the beginning of the twentieth century Spain's underdevelopment and poverty drove more than 6 million Spaniards to look for a better future elsewhere. This emigration was in two stages. In the first, between 1910 and 1935, 80 per cent of emigrants settled in Latin America. In the second stage, from 1960 to 1970, 75 per cent of emigrants travelled to the more industrially developed European countries.

The emigration of these two periods has created a legacy for the Spanish in terms of the formation of the identity of many of their population. The situation has also influenced, and continues to influence in part, a social policy that is focused upon improving the status of Spanish emigrants and the conditions for repatriation.

In the mid 1970s migration trends reversed. On the one hand, except for a small rise between 1981 and 1986, there was a gradual reduction in the numbers of people leaving Spain to live elsewhere. At the same time the number of Spaniards who had settled abroad and wanted to return to Spain increased. This trend was caused by the economic recession in Western countries, which led to most of them applying restrictions on new immigrants and encouraged the return of migrants to their home country.

It is interesting to note that according to the data from the Director General of Migration (1993), between 1982 and 1991 70 per cent of the 233,923 Spaniards that returned to Spain came from western European countries. In volume alone this migration flow constitutes one of the most significant demographic features in Spain's recent history.

Entry to Spain: a country of transit and destination

In parallel to Spaniards returning to their country of origin there has been the gradual growth of migrants into Spain. Between 1978 and 1988 the number of foreigners legally settling in Spain doubled and by 1992 nearly 400,000 people had settled in the country. Like other Mediterranean countries during the 1980s the concern in Spain was less with the issue raised by people leaving its shores and more with those migrating inwards.

However, Spain should not be characterized as being a country of immigration. There are still far more Spaniards living abroad than immigrants living in the country. As noted above almost 400,000 foreigners were living in Spain in 1992. The number of Spaniards living abroad in the same year was more than 1,500,000. That is, for every immigrant settled in Spain there were four Spaniards living abroad.

The official immigrant population of Spain has never been above 2.5 per cent of the total population. However, this figure is higher if illegal immigrants are added to this. Different sources provide different figures for this group. The Ministry of Labour and Social Security (1990) has estimated the number of illegal immigrants as being 170,000, while the Collective IOE (1989) gives an estimate of 400,000. If one takes the official figure and adds either of the two estimates the overall percentage of immigrants is small compared with those in other countries in the European Union. For example, in 1989 the figure for France was 6 per cent, Belgium and Germany 9 per cent, and in Luxembourg 26 per cent.

The fact that Spain has relatively few immigrants has had a corresponding minor impact upon its social structure, and this needs to be borne in mind when considering the nature of racism in the country. As Izquierdo (1992: 29) has stated, "the immigrant population in Spain is still small and has only recently established itself. This has meant that its influence on the Spanish social structure has been limited and the sociological understanding continually changing".

A number of different groups make up the immigrant population in Spain. Similarly there are different reasons for their settlement in the country. In 1975 those coming from European countries made up 62 per cent of the migrants, and in 1992 this figure was 50 per cent. Moreover, the majority of the Europeans are citizens of countries in the European Union. The figure for 1975 was 90 per cent and in 1992, 86 per cent. The second largest group comes from Central and South America. Immigrants from North America decreased in the period from 8 per cent of the total figure in 1975 to 4 per cent in 1992.

Foreigners coming from the Third World made up 8 per cent of immigrants in Spain in 1975. Between 1975 and 1992 there was a considerable increase in both the number and the percentage of people coming from Third World countries. The major increase has been in the number of those coming from Africa, in particular Morocco. In 1992 Moroccans formed 76 per cent, or 54,105, of those coming from Africa.

The study by the Collective IOE (1994) enables us to draw a correlation between the sociological profile and the geographical origin of those who have settled in Spain; it helps us distinguish between those who come from rich and poor countries, while examining the different socio-economical and cultural conditions of every group.

We can note for example that foreigners that migrate from developed countries basically form two different groups. The majority, from northern European countries, are pensioners who have chosen to live on the Mediterranean coast because of its favourable climatic conditions. According to official figures for 1992 only 29 per cent of the European inhabitants in Spain are economically active. These older immigrants are therefore a sizeable section within the larger non-economically active group. The economically active foreigners from developed countries are usually professionals from Europe, North America and Japan who have moved to Spain to work for multinational companies. Such companies are attracted to the areas of major economic and industrial growth, principally Madrid and Barcelona.

Those people who arrive from Third World countries come for different motives. In the majority of cases they are economic immigrants who are fleeing from poverty and a shortage of job opportunities in their own countries. They usually have few or no job qualifications and as a consequence their work opportunities are limited to employment demanding the use of heavy labour, low paid work, work in the black economy, domestic service, street selling, labouring in agriculture and the construction industry, and work in the hotel and catering industry. Many of the Third World immigrants experience problems of social marginalization. The situation has been described by the Collective IOE (1994: 88) in the following way.

In general the present situation favours the integration of immigrants from the European Community and those who are highly qualified. Those who experience problems are poorly qualified economic immigrants who find themselves exposed to the second labour market which is characterized by low pay, employment instability, lack of legal protection, and low trade union activity.

The reason for Spain's popularity as a country of destination for the economic immigrant can be explained, as it can for other countries receiving migrants, on the basis of economic and social factors. Inequality between nations has traditionally been countered by migration movements. In the case of Spain another important reason for immigration has been in operation. The attraction of Spain as a new social democratic country has led to many living in the nearby Magreb countries, and in particular Morocco, and to those with close linguistic, cultural and historical links, for example Latin America, wishing to participate in the economic prosperity of the country.

Spain's political, social and economic change coincided with the wider economic crisis of 1973 to 1985 which led to western European countries adopting restrictive migration policies. Another factor that was influential in the area of immigration was Spain's integration into the European Community. This gave Spain's southern coastline the role of the "Frontier of Europe". The country has had to adopt a strict control of migration flows from the south and in particular people from Third World countries who see Spain as a transit country or a country of destination.

There are therefore two influences upon the migration situation. On the one hand the hardening of the entry policies has increased the problems facing immigrants, particularly from the Third World, and stemmed their movement to Spain. On the other hand the process of the regularization of illegal immigrants, started in 1992, has revealed their needs and social problems which until then had been hidden. There has now been an attempt to improve a number of areas that affect such immigrants particularly in regard to housing, health, education, employment protection, and especially legal protection, improved salaries, and encouraging the membership of trade unions, as well as facilitating increased participation in the life of the country and attempting to assist the reunification of families.

Gypsies: foreigners in their own country

To understand the roots of racist attitudes and behaviour in Spanish society it is necessary to give specific attention to the gypsies. According to Giménez (1994) Spain's 500,000 gypsies can be described as "foreigners in their own land" because they suffer marginalization in their own country.

Gypsies first entered Spain in the fifteenth century and from then onwards began their marginalization and discrimination. In 1499 the Catholic kings introduced the first regulation of people of nomadic cultures by demanding that they choose between fixed settlement or exile. This persecution was increased by a succession of Spanish monarchs. In 1619 King Philip II ordered the removal of gypsy culture, in 1633 King Philip IV demanded that gypsies should be hunted with "iron and fire", and in 1695 King Charles II established the death penalty for those gypsies that continued their ambulant life style. However, early in the twentieth century it was recognized that gypsies belonged to groups that were in the greatest social danger and legislation was introduced recommending that the Civil Guard showed "scrupulous vigilance" over them.

At the time of writing the democratic constitution has led to gypsies being considered as Spanish citizens in their own right. Nevertheless, in general, Spanish society still views gypsies negatively and they continue to be marginalized. In the words of Calvo (1992a: 22):

> Gypsies are not only an ethnic group with a particular and cultural specificity, they are also a marginalized ethnic minority and maintain an inferior position in relation to the global society. It is in this structural relationship of dependency and exclusion that reside discriminated minorities.

No less significant are the conclusions of the Information on Racism in Europe (*European Parliament 1991*: 70–71) which stated that "in Spain the ethnic group that suffers the most discrimination is gypsies" and "the violent attacks on gypsy camps which occur now and then have their origins in local communities and are not part of a social movement".

The culmination of racist activity over the last five centuries has affected the collective view of gypsies. The new arguments put forward against gypsies include those that say they marginalize themselves. Another view is that gypsies are inclined to create a network of organized delinquency, particularly in relation to drugs.

Racism and xenophobia in Spanish society: a matter of concern

Although there exists within Spanish society a consistent and diverse number of episodes of ethnic intolerance, and in particular racism and xenophobia, the perception is that Spaniards are not racist and that in any case "the racists are the others" (Calvo 1989). This collective self-perception supports and justifies the response and attitude towards immigrants in Spanish society. What is clear is that significant immigration into Spain is a recent phenomenon and those that do settle in Spain are spread throughout the country with few opportunities for Spaniards and immigrants to live in close proximity.

A large number of the foreigners who settle in Spain come from western European countries and there is no strong feeling against them based upon their ethnic, racial or cultural background. In general, being in the main part renters or pensioners, their presence does not provoke negative reactions. On the contrary, Spaniards are either indifferent towards them or view their presence as positive because of the economic benefits they bring and the fact that they do not compete in the labour market.

Immigrants that come from Third World countries, however, are not integrated into areas occupied by either the western immigrants or the Spanish. Their presence in the country is almost invisible and explains in part the absence of an understanding by the Spaniards of this group of immigrants, and their feelings of rejection and the attitude of intolerance towards them. In the same way, it is easy to identify with positive stereotypes of tolerance and racial and cultural equality if one judges the racist and xenophobic actions as those of others, and those in other countries.

The distinction between foreigners who come from the Third World and those from developed countries is an important one in comprehending the logic of some of the xenophobic outbursts in Spain during the 1990s. According to the Collective IOE (1994: 1–13), Spanish public opinion "discriminates against the foreigners by classifying them into classes and responding negatively against some of them." That is, in general, the Spanish respond negatively towards those immigrants who can be classified as being socially marginalized because they reside in poverty, or have few labour skills, or exhibit anti-social behaviour. In this way the immigrants are not being discriminated against because of their race or different culture but because they are viewed as poor. On this theme Alvarez (1994: 43) talks of a "new racism" in which the "the exacerbation of xenophobia, the anxiety and the depreciation for those who are perceived as culturally (or socially) different or inferior, takes the place of biological racism".

The jolt from complacency in Spanish society, or in the opinion of Calvo (1992a) its awakening "from this narcissistic conceit which led us to believe that xenophobes were other people", started in 1992. On 13 November of that year, in an area on the periphery of Madrid, a black immigrant, Lucrecia Perez, from the Dominican Republic, was shot dead by an ultra-right-wing gang. This dramatic incident provoked a bitter realization that there existed in Spain a hidden racism, the victims being "poor" immigrants, many of them living illegally in the country, who existed in extreme marginal conditions. Lucrecia Perez was typical of such people. She left her husband and six-year-old daughter in the Dominican Republic, entering Spain via an illegal network of smuggling, expecting to find employment that would help get her family out of poverty. Although at the time of her death she was unemployed, Lucrecia, like other Dominican immigrants, had occasionally worked in domestic service, always without legal protection. Killed as she slept in the ruins of an abandoned discotheque, the murder of Lucrecia Perez was not the first such outbreak of violent xenophobia and racism this decade. In fact it was the culmination of a number of such incidents that occupied growing space in the media. Nevertheless the incident was to prove to be the most critical and led to an outcry by institutions and people against the violent racism that, it had been observed, was growing in different towns and villages throughout Europe.

Moreover, other similar incidents contributed to the theme of inequality and began to occupy political and social attention. Examples include the increase in local conflicts between gypsies and "poor" immigrants, the illegal entry of African immigrants across the Strait of Gibraltar with an undefined number of deaths at sea, the reorientation of Spanish politics to consider the problems of foreigners and migration, and a series of different surveys which were to highlight the growth in the rejection of foreigners.

Racist ideology does not receive any practical support from the major political forces in Spain and since the establishment of democracy ultra-right-wing parties have never surpassed 1 per cent of the total votes. However, there are certain skinhead gangs which perpetrate isolated violent acts against immigrants, those of other races, and marginal social groups such as homosexuals and beggars. In practice it is difficult to demonstrate the existence of a highly complex organization of gangs. The information we do have on such activities comes from the police and the Spanish Circle of European Friends. The periodical *Ford (Information on Racism*, European Community 1991: 70–71) has estimated that approximately 1,500 members of skinhead gangs in Spain are connected to similar organizations in other European countries.

Racism and social research

The new climate of concern about the relationship between the Spanish and immigrant groups has led to a drive by anthropologists, sociologists, psychologists and educators to analyse racism in more depth. In some cases this research has incorporated analytical perspectives which aim to generalize the results for the whole of the country. In other cases the research focuses on strategies and themes at a local and regional level. What follows are the most important conclusions drawn from the research.

In 1992 the government-supported Centre of Sociological

Investigation questioned Spaniards on their views on immigration and racism. The results were alarming:

- 48 per cent of respondents thought Spanish legislation was too generous in its permission for entry into the country by foreign labour.
- 61 per cent agreed with government measures to limit the entry of foreigners looking for work. The majority wanted to restrict the entry of Arabs and Africans.
- 27 per cent thought that illegal immigrants should be returned to their home country, while 59 per cent believed their situation should be regularized.
- 62 per cent believed that foreigners occupied jobs that could be undertaken by Spaniards, and 65 per cent thought their presence was unnecessary in the labour market.
- 52 per cent were of the opinion that there was a relationship between the settlement of foreigners and the selling of drugs.
- the groups that the respondents felt the greatest hostility towards were: gypsies (20 per cent); Arabs (13 per cent); Jews (9 per cent); blacks of African origin (8 per cent); North American blacks (7 per cent); Portuguese (6 per cent); and Filipinos and Hispanics (4 per cent).
- on a more positive note, 74 per cent respondents thought all foreigners should have the same rights as Spaniards, and 60 per cent of those interviewed wanted foreigners to have the vote.

Another survey conducted in the same year has provided valuable material, even though it refers only to data collected in Barcelona. The survey found that:

- of the most important issues concerning the respondents, "racial problems" appear 14th, being mentioned by only 0.7 per cent of those interviewed.
- overall 42 per cent of the respondents considered immigrants to be a problem. The figure for those respondents aged 45–54 years was 44 per cent, and for those between 12 and 24 years the figure was 33 per cent.
- while 27 per cent of those interviewed would like to have

closer links with immigrants (for example their children mar-
rying a foreigner), 47 per cent would not.
• the immigrants that respondents would not wish their son or
daughter to marry in order of rejection were: gypsies (40 per
cent); those from Magreb countries (37 per cent); Arabs (33
per cent); and "Negros" (30 per cent).

These data are especially revealing, showing tendencies confirmed by different investigations. However, it is important to
stress that Spaniards do not view themselves as racists or xenophobes when questioned directly. As De Miguel (1992) states,
"the social custom in pluralistic countries is not to be racist".Yet
when the question refers to concrete behaviour which centres
upon inter-ethnic or inter-racial relations the rejection of "the
others" is clear. According to Calvo (1992b) a radical explanation can be given for this, "... Spanish society says it is not racist
because it does not wish to kill black people, nor does it wish
them ill, but it also does not wish to get any closer to them."

Spanish young people's attitude towards immigration and racism is only a little different from that of the rest of the population.
In general they declare they are less racist and reject xenophobia.
Recent investigations indicate, however, that among young people there has been an increase in negative attitudes and perceptions towards foreigners and those of another race. The work by
Calvo demonstrates this change in attitude. Calvo carried out
investigations in 1987 (Calvo 1990) and 1993 (Calvo 1994) of
some 5,188 students aged from 14 to 19 years who were living
throughout Spain. When asked whether they would expel particular groups from the country 31 per cent of respondents in
1993 said they would remove gypsies (compared with 11 per cent
in 1987), 26 per cent would expel Arabs (11 per cent in 1987), 14
per cent black Africans (4 per cent in 1987), and 13 per cent Jews
(10 per cent in 1987). In the 1993 study, 46 per cent of those
interviewed considered the "white race superior to others".

A more recent study from the Centre for the Investigation of
Social Realities (CIRES 1994) offers similar if less problematic
data. The conclusions confirm that "only 6 per cent of citizens of

18 years and over can be considered to be real xenophobes or racists". Those aged between 18 and 24 years had a more tolerant view towards immigrants. All age groups rejected neo-Nazi groups, although a disturbing 25 per cent of respondents thought a party with such an ideology would be accepted in Spain.

Sociological studies of Spanish youth made since the International Year of Youth in 1985 make little reference to young people and the problem of racism. Those references that are to be found are short and located in sections dealing with the world of values, ideology and social attitudes. Those respondents that had an affinity with neo-Nazi groups rarely exceeded 2 per cent of those interviewed.

Politics and social legislation in Spain

As we have noted above, Spain became a social and constitutional state in 1978 with powers to promote social policy. In time it is thought Spain will become a social welfare state. By doing so it will overcome its long history of voluntarism that dates from the end of the nineteenth century until 1975. The stage that Spain is moving through is framed by different legal international treaties including the universal declaration of the rights of all people, international pacts covering economic, social and cultural rights, the European Charter; Spain's own Constitution, the 17 autonomous communities which form the basis of Spain's local government, and the autonomous laws of social services. Spain is therefore a decentralized state with central state administration, autonomous governments, and municipalities.

Although Spanish social policy is territorially varied it complies everywhere with the values of universality, equality, normalization, public responsibility, planning and co-ordination, participation, prevention and social integration. Essentially social policy is rooted in a public system of local social services which is overseen by the Ministry of Social Affairs, the autonomous communities, and the local authorities which exert control over the "Servicios Sociales" and the promotion of social obligations where there is a population of more than 20,000.

The formal development of state social policies is intended to stimulate and promote certain universal rights: health, education, social benefits, housing, culture, etc. At the same time the policies are aimed at addressing specific sectional concerns and intended to create equality of opportunities, personal and collective development, solidarity and social co-operation, and participation, especially in relation to people with disabilities, women, older people, youth, refugees, addicts, ethnic minorities and other groups.

The socio-economic crisis of the late 1980s and early 1990s has had an impact upon the availability and the scope of these social policy initiatives. The cuts in public expenditure, problems in the co-ordination of services, and limited resources for core social services have all added to the difficulties of meeting the above criteria. In short, in spite of progress, Spanish social policy has a number of weaknesses, disfunctions, shortages and limitations. One area of social policy that reflects these constraints is the approach to foreigners and those from ethnic minorities.

From emigration policies to immigration policies

Historically, the massive movement of Spaniards to other European countries and to Latin America from the end of the nineteenth century until the late 1960s focused the Spanish authorities' concern on an emigration policy directed at improving the personal and collective conditions of those Spaniards living abroad. After 1970 emigration waned and interest centred on internal migration within the country and immigration into Spain. In this relatively recent consideration of immigrants it was recognized that there was a lack of a clear immigration policy. Those policies that did exist dated from the nineteenth century when circumstances were very different. The 1978 Constitution was therefore a first attempt at addressing the issue.

Article 13 of the 1978 Constitution states that foreigners are entitled to fundamental liberties and rights. Article 14 conforms to the Universal Declaration on Human Rights, the International Pact on Civil Rights, and other international principles, stating that, "all Spaniards are equal before the law and no discrimination should take place because of birth, race, sex, religion, opinion or whatever other condition or personal circumstances". It is important to note that while the Constitution states that foreigners should enjoy the same freedoms and liberties as Spaniards, in practice there are specific laws that relate to immigrants (Sagarra i Trías 1991). These are part of the "law of foreigners" which was established in 1985.

On 7 November 1984 members of the Socialist government introduced to the Spanish Parliament a draft of a law that extended rights and liberties to foreigners. Passed as law in July 1985 it corrected the deficiencies of previous legislation while responding to the needs of those who wanted to settle in Spain. The new law, together with a plan for the "social integration of immigrants", aims to guarantee immigrants legal rights, to combat barriers which hinder their assimilation and entry into the labour market, and to mobilize society against xenophobia and racism. In this sense the law has made discrimination illegal. However, the growth of racist activity and xenophobia since 1985, and in particular in 1992 and the early part of 1993, has influenced the decision of the Parliamentary Committee of Justice and Interior to strengthen the laws for dealing with the aggravation of racism and xenophobia in a new penal code.

It has been thought that the absence of significant racist activity and xenophobia in the period 1985 to 1990 influenced and reflected Spanish society's response to immigration (De Lucas 1994). Critics argue that the underlying philosophy of the law has been the maintenance of public order rather than the welfare, liberties and rights of immigrants (Collective IOE 1993). The government, however, has insisted that it does not recognize the rights of immigrants while trying to equate their situation with Spaniards. In the opinion of the Executive, as stated at the Pleno del Congreso de Diputados in June 1990, "the technical complexities of the law together with the deficient administrative infrastructure have heavily hindered its correct application". According to the Government, the problems do not have their origins in the supposed repressive or "racist" character of the law, but in the ineffective management of immigration flows and the global negative views about foreigners.

On a more positive note, in 1996 legislation was introduced to assist immigrant families to reunite. These changes have been positively received by immigrant and other organizations in Spain.

The politics of youth policy

Spain has nearly 10 million people aged between 15 and 29 years, which is 25 per cent of the population. This number both in absolute terms and in relation to the rest of the population is without precedent in Spanish history. The view is that the significance of this group, as it is at the time of writing, is unlikely to be matched in future years.

The responsibility of the state and the different public administrations in relation to youth is formally regulated by Article 48 of the 1978 Spanish Constitution which declares that public authorities will "promote the conditions for free and effective participation of young people in relation to political, social, economical and cultural development". The 1992 Interministerial Plan for Youth and Childhood stressed the role of democratic pluralism in the participation and transition of young people into adult life by the means of economic integration.

Since 1982 the Central Administration has adopted various different measures aimed at integrating and promoting young people's participation in youth policy. The autonomous administrations have similarly developed policies for young people, particularly since the celebrations for the International Year of Youth in 1985. Because of the relationship of local authorities to the state, there are also opportunities for addressing social problems and needs, advancing an adequate policy for services and assisting in the process of youth participation.

In the third session of the Socialist Government in November 1991 the Spanish Council of Ministers presented a wide-ranging plan for the youth of the country. Entitled "Politics for the Generation of the 1990s" the plan tries to put into practice the principal recommendations made by the United Nations during the International Year of Youth. The purpose has been to establish a project aimed at the "autonomy and emancipation of every young person". The plan was reworked and refined by the Council of Ministers in November 1994.

When presented to the Government it was announced that the underlying purpose of the plan was to establish a central department to co-ordinate its youth policy, while encouraging other departments to address the needs of young people. The aim of the plan has been to share this political effort with youth itself through associations and youth councils. The plan brings together 244 measures intended to counter socio-political and economic inequality, and produce a structure that covers five main areas: education and employment, the quality of life, equal opportunities, participation and association, and international co-operation.

The plan's editorial committee stated that the rejection of racism and xenophobia were to be the primary aim for the next few years. They state that there is a good deal of racist activity in Europe, particularly – because of unemployment and industrial change – among the most impoverished members of the European Community. However, the committee also states that forces against racism and the discrimination of immigrants, refugees or people from ethnic groups are in the ascendancy.

Initiatives and experiences in youth work

The rise of racist, xenophobic and violent attitudes and behaviour in Spain during the 1990s has brought to the fore the need for young people to adopt an active programme to combat the problem. There is a particular need to encourage young Spaniards to consider and act upon initiatives that promote and safeguard human rights and respect and mutual tolerance in the context of a pluralistic and democratic society. This requires a collective effort involving all those organizations and institutions linked with young people, associated youth movements and, more importantly, every young person.

The Interministerial Commission for Young People and Children in its Integral Plan for Youth has rejected racist and xenophobic activity and has stated the need to promote and integrate members of ethnic minorities from adolescence. The plan advocates two specific measures:

(a) The schooling of gypsy youth. This involves the Ministry of Education and Science in the integration of gypsy young people in ordinary schools.

(b) The design and execution of preventive measures against the discrimination of young people because of their ethnicity or religion. The purpose is to promote a climate of friendship and understanding. To do this the plan advocates the launching of an informative campaign aimed at explaining the customs of young people from ethnic groups and the problems they face. It is felt this will promote solidarity with non-Spaniards.

To assist this the Youth Institute has, since 1992, assumed a campaign for combating racism. The campaign has stressed the pluralist nature of Spanish society and the need for the contribution of different opinions and the value of a variety of approaches and organizations particularly in the areas of education, leisure, political action, socio-cultural events, communal radio and so forth. The campaign appears to have been successful and there are now more than 400 internal and external activities and

83

programmes which involve approximately 200,000 young people between the ages of 16 and 24 years.

The plan has been complemented by a campaign for democracy in equalness which has been financed since 1983 by the Ministry of Social Affairs with 0.5 per cent of the raised income tax. The aim of the campaign has been to promote respect for differences and the equality of all people of whatever ethnicity, nation of origin, disability or sexuality. The campaign has aimed at achieving a real debate on the issue of equality, and recognizing plurality and tolerance as positive values in assisting integration in society.

The initiative that has brought about the greatest amount of change is that launched in April 1993 to combat intolerance in young people. The purpose of the initiative is to address the problem of intolerance among young people towards minority groups. The initiative is based on a civic process of stimulating within Spanish society the principles of solidarity, of living in harmony, and of social equality. The intention has also been to establish a strategy aimed at diffusing racism, to establish a project that involves meetings and activities that engage the work of games instructors and youth workers, the publication of teaching material aimed at involving schools and associations and the involvement of immigrants, refugees and ethnic minorities in cultural activities and events that focus on their rights and encourages their integration into Spanish society.

Nearly 20 associations, groups and non-governmental organizations, as well as local affiliations, are involved in the project. They all conform to what is considered to be the most important initiative in Spain to establish a social base aimed at eradicating racism, xenophobia and the resulting violence. The initiative's motto is "Only one race, the human race".

As well as the high profile campaigns described above there has been a number of progressive initiatives established since the beginning of the 1990s directed at working with young people in the struggle against racism and xenophobia. Some of these have been linked with work at an international level. Such initiatives have included:

- The Young Person's Manifesto against Racism which is subscribed to by 75 youth organizations and youth councils and which celebrated on 21 March 1993 the International Day Against Racism. The manifesto states that Spain is part of a multi-ethnic, multinational Europe and needs to work towards the eradication of xenophobia and racism throughout the world.
- The Spanish Committee of the European Campaign against Racism, Xenophobia and Intolerance. This was created on 27 July 1994 and co-ordinated the Spanish contribution to the United Nations 1995 International Year of Tolerance.
- The establishment of various courses and seminars with themes related to immigration, racism and the politics of social integration within programmes at universities in Verano. These universities have held conferences for young people from all over Spain.
- An international meeting held in 1993 under the motto "Combat Racism" which aimed to encourage young people to reflect upon, debate and condemn the segregation and marginalization of racial minorities, and to appreciate the value of cultural riches.
- The celebration of diverse artistic, cultural and creative happenings in numerous Spanish villages and towns. Since 1993 such celebrations have included inter-ethnic meetings, concerts, summer camps, exhibitions of posters and photographs, literary competitions, a variety of festivals, a cultural week and so forth.

For those events that are targeted at children and young people there has been a growing development of multicultural and intercultural education programmes. The reform of the Spanish education system has led to changes in the training of teachers and in the production of didactic materials that focus on ethnic minorities, racism, xenophobia and cultural pluralism. The first initiative has been to produce, in collaboration with the publishing company Editorial Popular, materials that use these themes. This work has been financially supported by the Ministry of Social Affairs.

Conclusion

In this chapter we have argued that Spain is only now beginning to confront the problems raised by immigration. Although it is unwise to generalize in the context of European countries, it is possible to state that in regard to racism and xenophobia the situation in Spain is little different from that experienced in other European countries. Nevertheless, it is clear that after many years where the dominant feature was Spaniards emigrating, the country has now become one of transit and destination for foreigners. As a consequence, the traditional politics of emigration have been superseded by the politics of immigration. The restrictions on immigration have led to a good deal of political and social questioning.

We have noted that the legislative, social and economic initiatives relating to immigration are far from desirable. Not only is there a divergence between expectations and reality, there is also a recognition that more attention needs to be placed on key areas including the elimination of racist and xenophobic perceptions, conduct and attitudes, a change in the individual and collective mentality about cultural characteristics and different identities, encouraging communal solidarity and social integration in areas of economic deprivation, and stimulating the full integration of immigrants into Spanish society, particularly in the fields of employment, education, health and leisure.

The complexity of the situation makes it difficult to predict the future. What needs to be done is: prepare young people to take on these commitments and responsibilities in their daily life; promote initiatives which encourage the integration and social cohesion of all people living in Spain; face the challenge of a civic process in which mutual respect and living in harmony is encouraged; and support the recognition that diversity is one of the best heritages mankind has given us.

The tasks outlined above are ones which Spanish youth policy appears equipped to meet. More importantly there is a broad range of collectives which encourage cultural pluralism and reject racism and xenophobia. The aim is that these policy and practice initiatives will form part of a common challenge throughout Spanish society.

References and further reading

Abad, L., A. Cucò, A. Izquierdo (eds), 1993. *Inmigración, pluralismo y tolerancia*. Madrid: Popular/Jóvenes contra la Intolerancia.

Ajuntament de Barcelona 1992. *Actituds dels barcelonis envers els inmigrants provinents d'altres cultures*. Barcelona: Consell Municipal de Benestar Social.Á

Alvarez, I. 1994. "Los retos de la inmigración". Los retos de la inmigración. Racismo y pluriculturalidad. See Colectivo IOE 1994. Madrid: Talasa.

Arias, I, y Otros 1993. *Racimo y xenofobia: búsqueda de las raices*. Madrid: Fundación Rich.

Cánovas, F. y Otros 1984. Politicas de Juventud y Administraciones Públicas. In *Politicas de Juventud y Administraciones Públicas*, Ministerio de Cultura. Madrid: Ministerio de Cultura.

Calvo, R. y Otros (ed.) 1984. *Educa para la tolerancia*. Madrid: Popular/Jóvenes contra la Intolerancia.

Calvo, T. (ed.) 1989. *Los racistas son los otros*. Madrid: Popular.

Calvo, T. 1990. *España racista? Voces payas sobre los gitanos*. Barcelona: Anthropos.

Calvo, T. 1992a. "El rostro de la ..." *El Pais*, 22 November, 2.

Calvo, T. 1992b. En referencia de C. Diaz Los adolescentes españoles. *El Pais*, 2 January, 16.

Calvo, T. 1994. *El racismo que viene*. Madrid: Tecnos.

CIRES 1994. *Actitudes hacia los inmigrantes*. Madrid: CIRES.

Colectivo IOE 1989. España, frontera sur de Europa. *Documentación Social*, 77, 101–9.

Colectivo IOE 1993. La inmigración en España: principales tendencias.

In *La inmigración*, Colectivo IOE, A. Y. Martínez, M. L. Sànchez. Conversaciones 92. Popular, Madrid, 29–122.

Colectivo IOE 1994. La inmigración extranjera en España: sus caracteristicas diferenciadoras en el contexto europeo. In *Los retos de la inmigración. Racismo y Pluriculturalidad.* J. Contreras (ed.), Madrid: Talasa.

Comisión Interministerial para la Juventud y la Infancia 1992. Plan Integral de Juventud. Politicas para la generación de los 90. Madrid: Instituto de la Juventud/Ministerio de Asuntos Sociales.

Consejo de la Juventud de España 1991. *Bases para una politica de juventud.* Madrid: Consejo de la Juventud de España.

De Lucas, J. 1994. *Europa, convivir con la diferencia?: Racismo, nacionalismo y derechos de las minorias* (2nd edition). Madrid: Tecnos.

De Miguel, A. 1992. *La sociedad española, 1992–93.* Madrid: Alianza edt.

Del Campo, S. 1992. Sobre el racismo y la xenofobia. *Cuenta y Razón del Pensamiento Actual*, 73–4.

Dirección General de Migraciones 1993. Anuario de Migraciones 1993. Madrid: Ministerio de Trabajo y Seguridad Social.

European Parliament 1991. *Information on Racism in Europe* 70–71. Madrid: Ministerio de Asuntos Sociales.

Elzo, J. 1994. *Jóvenes españoles, 1994.* Madrid: Ediciones SM.

Giménez, A. 1994. Extranjeros en su propia tierra: los gitanos. In *Extranjeros en el paraiso.* Barcelona: Virus Edt.

Herrera, M. 1993. Inmigración, xenofobia y racismo en España, *Sal Terrae*, **43**, 55–71.

Higuera, G. 1992. Xenofobia y racismo. *Revista de Fomento Social*, **47**, 169–83.

Ibarra, E. 1994. Jóvenes contra la intolerancia... *Documentación Social*, **95**, 199–208.

Izquierdo, A. 1992. España como pais de acogida. *Cuenta y Razón del Pensamiento Actual*, 73–4, 28–35.

Izquierdo, A. 1993. Politica e inmigración en la España de 1992. In *Integración, Pluralismo y tolerancia.* L. Abab, A. Cucó, A. Izquierdo, 87–124. Madrid: Popular/Jóvenes contra la Intolerancia.

Martin Serrano, M. 1991. Cultura gitana y cambio social. Actas de las III Jornadas de Psicologia de la Intervención Social. Madrid: Ministerio de Asuntos Sociales, Madrid.

Ministry of Labour and Social Security 1990. *Anuario de migraciones.* Madrid: Direccion General de Migraciones del Ministerio de Trabajo y Seguridad Social.

Navarro, M. M. J. Mateo, 1993. *Informe Juventud en España 1992, Injuve.* Madrid: Ministerio de Asuntos Sociales.

REFERENCES AND FURTHER READING

Sagarra i Trías, E. 1991. *Los Derechos fundamentales y las libertades públicas de los extranjeros en España. Protección jurisdiccional y garantias.* Barcelona: Bosch Edt.

Tamames, R. 1994. *Introducción a la economia española.* Madrid: Alianza Edt.

Tiempo y Paz 1992. monográfico "Racismo y xenofobia", 23.

Zarraga, J. L. 1989. *Informe Juventud en España, 1988.* Injuve. Madrid: Ministerio de Asuntos Sociales.

[references, faded/mirror-image and illegible]

5

Racism in the new Germany: examining the causes, looking for answers

Rudolf Leiprecht, Lena Inowlocki, Athanasios Marvakism and Jürgen Novak

Introduction

Racial violence has escalated alarmingly in the new Germany. For the year 1993, official statistics from the Federal Criminal Investigation Agency indicate a total of 6,721 racial crimes and violent offences. These include attacks on refugee accommodation and the homes of immigrants, attacks on people, including killings, wilful damage to property, threats, insults and slander, and propaganda offences. It is a sad story to tell when we are discussing the societal causes of such violence and the role of young people. It is even sadder because the counter movement against racism only gained a significant societal impact after the murder of Turkish migrants in the town of Mölln in November 1992. The protest against attacks on foreigners was expressed in an advertising campaign, in candlelit chains of several hundred thousand participants, and in large demonstrations in all federal states. Similarly, *Mahnwachen* (symbol guarding) and telephone chains were organized to protect homes of asylum-seeking refugees. Meanwhile, some political groups demanded the introduction of dual citizenship for refugees. It would be preferable to be able to report an increase in this counter movement. Our task however, is to provide an analytical overview and, as will be noted, negative aspects are continuing to determine developments in the new Germany.

Racial violence and the power of labelling

Between 1987 and 1990 the cases of recorded racial violence numbered 250. In the second half of 1991, however, this figure had significantly increased and in the whole of that year 2,427 cases were reported. A year later another enormous increase took place with 6,336 cases registered. Figures remain high, and in 1994, 3,491 racial crimes were reported (Bundes-Kriminalamt 1995).

Examination of these figures indicate that in absolute terms there is more racial crime and violence in *West* Germany. If we take into account the number of inhabitants in the federal states, then the whole picture is changed negatively in regard to *East* Germany. What is important, however, is that the escalation of racial violence is a problem in both West and East Germany. Such a statement is not intended to be superficial, but to counter the view held by many politicians and sections of the mass media who have tried to persuade the public that racism is predominantly a phenomenon of East Germany (Leiprecht 1992).

Breaking down criminal statistics into age groups we note that 75 per cent of the suspected persons, who were investigated because of criminal and violent offences, were under 20 years of age (Willems et al. 1993: 16). So, is racism in Germany mainly a youth problem?

This would be an extremely narrow point of view. Looking at the results from opinion polls, we note that young people are generally more tolerant towards immigrants and refugees than comparative groups of adults (Wahl 1993: 15). Moreover, young people do not live in a vacuum but are shaped by particular societal circumstances. As stated by Wahl "the political atmosphere in Germany of the nineties, the opinion shapers and the applauding audiences of mature adults" should not be excluded from our perception (Wahl 1993: 5).

However, a limited view can be observed in many public discussions. The racist activity is thought to derive from violent or unemployed young people who are poorly educated and unsure of themselves. These young people are thought to be disadvantaged and living at the margins of society. With this "power of labelling" the problem is more or less clearly limited to a particular social sphere and to a particular group of people. Thus professionals such as politicians, journalists and trade union officials, as well as teachers and social scientists, have condoned their own responsibility and argue that we are dealing with a youth problem, or a problem at the margins of society (Rommelspacher 1992: 82).

Changes in the discussion of the term right-wing extremism

Since the late 1980s there has been an increase in discussions on racism in Germany. Previously the problem was denied or trivialized or, like in the former GDR, ascribed to the enemy of the system. During the early development of the old Federal Republic little research on neo-fascism and right-wing extremism was carried out (Paul & Schoßig 1979; Meyer & Rabe 1979). Research grew from concern with the election success of the right-wing extremist party of the National Democrats (NDP) at the end of the 1960s, the increase in members of right-wing extremist groups and youth organizations, and with the increasing militance of right-extremism. Furthermore, this research originated in the aftermath of the anti-authoritarian regimes (For example, see the discussions about theories of fascism in Kühnl 1974). In these works the term fascism and the continuation of fascism in democratic societies were examined. Auschwitz and the extermination of the Jews were recognized as the important indicators of a

93

specific German fascism. However, contemporary anti-Semitism and inner societal racism were given sparse attention.

Therefore the more informed discussion on the phenomenon of racism is quite recent and the discussion of terms mirrors what is taking place in other countries. The debate in Germany has been informed among others by the translated works of Robert Miles (in German in 1989 and 1991) and drew the attention to the term "racialization" in the (old) Federal Republic of Germany.

Germany as an immigrant society

Historically, migration or migratory movements within the geographical area which now accommodates the German nation state have been the norm rather than the exception. In the light of this, the claim that the German people (*Volk*) have a "naturally originating" homogenous character becomes absurd. In the literature, we find many examples of migration both previous to and during contemporary times (Engelmann 1984; Page Moch 1992; Bade 1993; Herbert 1986). An example of migration dates from the early post-war years, when between 1945 and 1950 almost 12 million people, exiles from Eastern Europe and displaced persons, fled westwards into the territories occupied by western powers which later became the Federal Republic. In addition three million East German citizens fled and settled in West Germany before the wall was built in 1961.

This example in particular shows how large numbers of immigrants can be integrated despite poor economic conditions such as were present in Germany during the post-war period. The fact that these refugees were immediately granted citizenship rights, and that their immigration was supported by the main political groups, undoubtedly contributed to their social integration. The example also shows how inappropriate it would be to look exclusively at the number of immigrants (cf. Bade 1985).

In recent years the numbers of immigrants have, unfortunately, been used as a device in the political discussion. For example, at the end of the 1980s, when the number of people applying for political asylum in Germany clearly increased and, at the same time, more and more so-called *Aussiedler* (Eastern European "ethnic Germans") made use of their right to become German citizens, refugees were increasingly separated into categories of "good" and "bad" in the dominant political discourse and the media.[1] Whereas there were many appeals from politicians and advertising campaigns for a warm welcome for the *Aussiedler*, the group that had applied for asylum were viewed as a matter of "grave and serious concern". One newcomer was to be welcomed as a "fellow German", the other was presented as an "economic refugee" who had come for self-interested motives and was nothing but a burden on the German tax payer. Whereas one was to be considered a "useful enrichment" to the Republic, the other was associated with images such as "ruin" and "danger". The rise in the number of applicants for asylum was presented in reports which were outright sensationalist and intended to shock (cd. Leiprecht 1990: 215ff.).[2] Empirical investigations have shown that many young people took up the negative comments of politicians and the media whilst generalizing and extending them to all groups which they perceived as "foreigners", thus including "Aussiedler" and migrant workers (Leiprecht 1990: 365).

That the Federal Republic is a country of immigration, while admittedly one which wishes to recognize this neither politically nor institutionally, is demonstrated by examining the population statistics. Most interesting is not that the new FRG had 6.8 million registered "foreigners" in 1993, which is 8.3 per cent of the total population, but rather that approximately 60 per cent of this group had already been in Germany for more than eight years and therefore were hardly "foreigners" (Statistisches Bundesamt [Federal Department of Statistics] 1995). Despite an increase in total population in the new republic (65 million West Germans and 16 million East Germans), the proportion of foreigners declined after the unification of the FRG and the GDR because the former GDR had very few immigrants. Not only were immigrant numbers extremely low in the GDR (1.2 per cent in 1990), they have remained so in the new states (1 per cent in 1992).

This last figure deserves further attention because states that have few foreigners exhibit a great deal of extremely aggressive forms of racism. Therefore, the often heard formula "lots of immigration equals lots of racism" should be viewed with great scepticism. The effect of this equation contributes to making the targets of racism themselves responsible for racism.

Nevertheless, it cannot be denied that a large number of people entering at once can cause problems, even when the country is prosperous. The federal and state governments, however, chiefly leave solutions to practical problems such as accommodation to local politicians (cf. Willems et al., 1993: 120). Unfortunately, migration in the 1990s has not, as a rule, been seen as a challenge to ensure a better spread of refugees within Europe and to assist in the new long-term goal of securing international solidarity as part of the fundamental reform of the world economy. In the short term the influx has placed demands on administrators and politicians who must provide people with satisfactory accommodation. Unfortunately, the attitude of hostility has been most prominent.

Ethnic inequality

Even though the children of immigrants make up 20 per cent of young people in places such as the state of Baden-Württemberg, research among young people in Germany generally indicates no particular attention to this group.[3] Such a "blind spot" has a particular overtone given that in Germany there is still a clear correlation between ethnicity and poor social conditions. Ethnic inequality can be shown by means of diverse indicators such as immigrants' exclusion from the political process and their

ETHNIC INEQUALITY

inferior legal position. For example, involvement in the political process is limited by the aliens law (*Ausländergesetz*), and drawing social security can be grounds for expulsion.

Ethnic minority groups are excluded from political participation at all levels of the political system. They have no voting rights, and do not have the right to stand for election to a local government, a state parliament (*Landtag*), or the Federal Parliament (*Bundestag*). In 1992 the state parliament of the city of Hamburg decided to give voting rights to non-German citizens. However, a successful legal action to block this was brought to the Federal Constitutional Court by a number of conservatives. The judges ruled that within the German constitution the only legitimate basis for democratic power is German citizenship. They concluded that voting rights could not be granted to non-citizens. Following from this, in April 1994 a majority in the Federal Parliament voted against the introduction of dual citizenship.

Another indicator of inequality is the labour market. Among immigrants there is a higher proportion of unskilled and semi-skilled workers (cf. Seifert 1992, 1993). Research regularly establishes the development of an "ethnically biased lower class" (Gillmeister & Kurthen 1989: 305). Among the unemployed there are still disproportionately large numbers of immigrants. For example, in Hamburg in 1990 immigrants made up 7.5 per cent of the employed but 14.8 per cent of those out of work. This is often attributed to their lower qualifications. However, immigrants are also clearly over-represented amongst the better-qualified unemployed (cf. Räthzel & Sarica 1994: 23).

School is often a source of major problems for the children of immigrants. In Berlin approximately 24 per cent of this group leave school without a completed qualification; among Germans of their age the proportion is 10 per cent. Since the end of the 1980s, however, there have been signs of a slightly improved structural social integration of immigrants. Looking at the percentage of young people from immigrant families in vocational training there appears to be an increase. In 1991 7.6 per cent were in training compared (in the previous FRG) to 2.9 per cent in 1985. However, during the same period the proportion of immigrant young people in the age group 15–18 years increased from 7.9 per cent to 15.6 per cent (Tränhardt et al. 1995). Among young people, the relationship between ethnicity and unfavourable social situations seems to have weakened. For example, there is an increasing participation of "non-German" youth in the vocational training system. However, these figures should be treated with care. "Non-German" youth are located in particular vocations, for example they are over-represented in trades and are almost completely excluded from public administration (Granato 1995: 12).

Overall, the situation for immigrants has been described as a

legal system which makes them insecure and discriminates against them, an educational and vocational system in which little consideration is given to their needs and circumstances, as well as minimal demand for their specific abilities (e.g. bilingualism), non-recognition of qualifications they have gained in their countries of origin, etc. . . . from the outset these made for poorer preconditions for the labour market (Räthzel & Sarica, 1994: 27–8).

Racism in the former FRG and GDR

The escalation of violence in Germany during the second half of 1991 has a long history which we now briefly discuss.

Before German unification a report from the European Parliament warned of the extent of racism and xenophobia in the old FRG (Ford 1990). This situation was supported at the economic-legal level by the systematic discrimination against immigrant workers (Castels 1987; Kühne 1987; Osterkamp 1989). The different treatment of German and immigrant workers had intensified over a number of years. For example, in November 1973, on instruction from the Federal Institute of Labour, the law of labour promotion led to unemployed Germans being given preferences for jobs over foreign workers (Katsoulis 1984: 192). This different treatment of Germans and immigrants has been protected and administered by a number of institutions. Such institutional discrimination supports and reproduces the tendency in the population to accept inferiority. A further example of this development can be found at the political level. In the West German election campaigns of the 1980s and the early 1990s the political parties frequently talked of "flooding", "a breach in the dam", "the boat is full", "a time bomb", "an extensive blaze", etc. in regard to immigrants (Ruhrmann 1987; Uihlein & Weber 1989: 15).

On the scientific ideological level a similar discourse about what is "national" can be observed. Historians such as Fest, Nolte, Hillgruber and Stürmer made an effort in the so-called "historians dispute" to revise German history by introducing the word "normalization". In this sense the political scientist and philosopher Willms characterized the moral condemnation of the crimes of German fascism as "a weapon to try permanently to keep the Germans as a nation in subjection" (Klönne 1987).

In the former GDR, observers of right-wing extremism have been concerned about the growth of racism since the attack by skinheads at a meeting in the East Berlin Zion Church in October 1987. This attack was to lead to an increase in right-wing activity. Edith Broszinsky-Schwabe from the East Berlin Humboldt University emphasizes that in the former GDR racism was

> latent, but the press and the propaganda concealed the truth because it did not fit in with the image of the GDR. Acts of violence against foreigners were hardly ever prosecuted by the police (Brozinsky-Schwabe 1990: 35).

These findings, however, were never allowed to be published. Different attempts at an explanation by GDR authors can be pieced together to form a general picture. For example, the former GDR citizen Konrad Weiss explains that the increase of right-wing activity or ideologies were well suited to daily life in the GDR.

> The right wing enjoys an increasing acceptance in working and education groups and to the unpolitical observer righ-wing extremists appear as industrious, tidy, and disciplined young citizens (Weiß 1989: 43).

The social scientist Hermann Langer from Rostock believes "the increasing crisis of the real existing socialism" is due to a number of reasons.

> The incompetence of the (communist) SED leadership to solve serious problems and the attempt to cover it up by reports of success and doctored statistics led to an increasing decline of values. The retreat of the majority into the private niches created a vacuum. Many young people reacted to the hypocrisy of the parental home, regimentation in schools, and the senseless work in the communist youth organization FDJ. They developed a sort of contraposition, supporting neo-Nazi slogans (Langer 1991:93).

Wolfgang Brück from the Youth Institute in Leipzig refers to "the artefact socialism in the colours of the GDR" as an expression of nationalistic superiority and with it a more or less subliminal reaction towards the supposedly inefficient Poles and Romanians (Brück 1988).

National Socialism and racism

Racism in Germany has long been exclusively regarded in connection with "fascism in power", i.e. National Socialism. The democratic FRG has defined itself as "totally different". This division has made it difficult and even incomprehensible why and how millions of "normal" and "ordinary" citizens of the democratic Weimar Republic helped National Socialism to come to power (see Kalpaka & Räthzel 1990).

In the former GDR an understanding of the role of everyday life in the creation of National Socialism was ignored. Instead a shortened thesis of monopoly capitalism, which had helped fascism come to power, became the state doctrine. As a result, all citizens of the "socialistic" GDR could be declared anti-fascists. When fascism and racism were identified they were thought to be the result of hostile manipulation and the impact of the capitalist West. The almost smooth transition from fascism in power to post-war Stalinism in the GDR was supported by many people who were accustomed to subordination, obedience and trust in authority. Criticism was, therefore, never considered. This formally prescribed anti-fascism "from above" was, in many people's view, very superficial. The outcome has been that a critical debate on the history of National Socialism, and the actual dangers from "the extreme right" are rejected by many young people in Germany because of their experiences of the empty phrases of the authoritarian GDR-socialism (Schubarth & Schmidt 1992; Langer 1991).

Similarly, in the old FRG there was no real understanding of fascism. The initial attempts of the allies to remove fascism were undercut when, at the beginning of the cold war, many National Socialist judges, civil servants, professors and doctors regained prominent positions in the FRG. The post-war years were characterized by a silence about the past. Economic wealth had absolute priority. Moreover the "new" opponent – the communist bloc in the East – was also in some senses the "old" opponent.

Towards the end of the 1960s the anti-authoritarian student, apprentice and high-school student movement revolted against this silence. A number of them "exposed" their parents – even though in a self-righteous way – as fascists. While the parents were defined as culprits, the sons and daughters believed themselves victims of the National Socialistic past and of post-war capitalism. The struggle against fascism and right-wing governments led to international solidarity, especially with liberation movements (e.g. during the Vietnam war). However, anti-American and anti-Jewish sentiments were often indirectly supported by these movements.

The anti-authoritarian movements changed in part the face of FRG society and a clear tension developed between the public discussions and the continual "private silence" in the vast majority of families. Nevertheless this silence is not a private affair. It is related to the general inability in German society to reflect critically on National Socialism. Involvement in the murderous system is minimized by the older generation, as well as by their family members (Rosenthal 1992). Right-extremist group ideology turns the defensive denial into offensive claims and since the late 1970s the denial of the holocaust has provided right-wing groups with an effective instrument of recruitment. Interviews with members of right-wing extremist youth groups indicate that the rhetoric of denial has been a strong mobilizing factor (Inowlocki 1992). This begins with the "insight" transmitted through older group leaders and, significantly, through proselytizers of the war generation that "nothing" happened to the Jews and that Germans are the real victims. With rhetorical proficiency in group ideology comes the "discovery" that claims can be made about historical and social reality, while new recruits might believe that with the denial "truth" becomes irrelevant. The power to claim what is "history" has profound effects in biographical terms too. Personal history is rewritten as group members talk themselves into "historical" and "national" relevance.

Other research based on narrative interviews and biographical analysis similarly shows how young right extremists rely on the general lack of reflection on National Socialism as well as, in particular, on the ongoing identification by some members of the older generation with National Socialism (Schiebel 1992). However, mainstream research is based on the hypothesis that only present social problems are relevant for an understanding of right-wing extremist orientations of youth (Heitmeyer 1987, Heitmeyer et al. 1992). This view excludes a reconstruction of how "social problems" have become defined and generally accepted; how, for example, in the critical situation of Germany during and after unification, a relapse could occur into patterns of interpretation of being invaded and threatened by "foreigners". In place of an analysis of the symbolic, historical dimensions of the hatred and persecution of foreigners, "real" problems caused by "too many" foreigners are assumed. It is overlooked how the different generations have been shaped by the experience and history of National Socialism.

The new Federal Republic of Germany

In the autumn of 1990 the unification of the FRG and GDR created a new society. Although unification was established by constitutional law, the experience was an emotional one for its citizens. In all, five new federal states were added. However, the economic and social aspects of unification proved to be more difficult than most politicians had previously thought and claimed.

In the new federal states problems of transformation quickly emerged and have demanded a fundamentally new way for people to address social relations, their relationship to the state bureaucracy, and in their political action. In the former GDR there have been massive cutbacks in youth work. At the same time the level of youth unemployment in the new federal states far exceeds that of West Germany. Former class comrades and colleagues are increasingly competitors in the market for meagre trainee posts, apprenticeships and jobs. The East German youth researcher Schubarth states: "the social upheaval not only creates anomie and disintegration, it also destroys the old support systems, while new support systems for the future have yet to be developed" (Schubarth 1993: 258). Schubarth concludes that there is no automatic correlation between worsening social and economic circumstances and increasing extreme right-wing activity. The main factor is the legacy of the authoritarian communist SED state. This involves the collective interpretation of problems in the new federal states,

> the experiences with an authoritarian state, with undemocratic societal structures, with intolerance, intimidations, repressions and violence have promoted the development of authoritarian undemocratic ways of thinking and behaviour (Schubarth 1993: 259).

A characteristic of unification experienced on both sides of Germany was its relatively short process. Unification was primarily "the side product of unexpected developments outside of Germany" (Hobsbawm 1991: 203). After unification, efforts were made in the public discourse to create a common consciousness for the new national state. This discourse of "national" can also be seen as a determining factor in the development of increasing right-wing activity (Held et al. 1995a: 4).

The selected strategies in the creation of an all-embracing national consciousness were characterized by specific contradictions. In the return to a common German history the positive elements are usually emphasized, often excluding dealing with the more recent history of National Socialism. While efforts were made to create a national common symbol, the effect has been to create a social rift between East and West Germany with increasing gestures of superiority by the West Germans towards East Germans. In a renewed sharpening of the asylum discussion, concepts of the "enemy" and the danger "from outside" have been constructed. At the same time, because of sensitivity to international relations, the authorities condemned violence towards refugees provoked by the asylum discussion.

In their analysis of the media, several linguistic scientists have pointed to a newly intensified and extremely aggressive view of immigrants and refugees as the social problem (see Gerhard 1991; Huhnke 1993; Jäger et al. 1993; Loose 1993). A large section of the established politics and the media have created a panic in public opinion. One example of many is a letter sent during the summer of 1991 by Volker Rühe, the then general secretary of the ruling Christian Democratic Union (CDU) to all local and communal functionaries. In his letter, Rühe announced that asylum legislation and immigration should be made election campaign issues. Forms were included for "individual" communal complaints about asylum-seeking refugees – only the town name had to be filled in. Another example is the headline in bold letters of the widely read *BILD-Zeitung* of 3 August 1991, quoting the federal secretary of the interior, Schäuble: "Now it's enough with asylants". A few days later, a daily series of articles entitled: "Asylants in Germany. Who should pay?" was advertised on large posters all over the Federal Republic.

The established politicians appeared helpless towards the violence. This had the effect of stimulating violence. In the analysis of escalating racial violence a research group from Trier claimed that "the success of the violent criminals represented a central mobilising factor in the further development of crimes of violence and criminal offences" (Willems et al. 1993: 9). To these factors one must add the apparent failure of the police and the public prosecutor's office which allowed such behaviour to continue, as well as the political success of right-wing extremist groups. Right-wing groups have interpreted this lack of action as a sign from the established politics that political changes, including constitutional amendments, could be forced through by violent action in the streets and by destroying houses where immigrants and refugees lived. "The dull heart could experience: the problem of hatred of foreigners is the foreigners themselves" (Habermas 1993: 166).

Some results of recent empirical youth research

Research indicates that many young violent racist offenders see themselves as active agents who translate the words of politicians into "clear acts". While "those above" do the talking, these young people interpret their violence as executing the political discourse into "acts of consequence" (see also Quinkert & Jäger 1991). At the same time, research makes clear that only a small minority of young people have a complete right-wing conception of the world. The political attitude of most young people seems to be contradictory and inconsistent. This is supported by the results of a research project in Tübingen in which a comparative opinion poll among young trainees from East and West Germany was carried out (Held et al. 1995b). In certain respects the attitude of these young people reflects the contradictions of the dominant policy towards "foreigners" – for example, to behave "friendly to foreigners" and at the same time to act with hostility towards foreigners. A generalized political trend since the mid 1980s is that young people move to the "right" as they become older. At the time of writing, however, it seems that the younger the person, the more likely he will hold right-wing views.

Political parties and trade unions argue that it is the worsening of life chances that is responsible for the increasing shift to the right. There is no doubt that the economic crisis has had a determining influence on young people's life chances in both East and West Germany. The Tübingen research was analysed to see if aspects of life chances correlated in any way with political orientations. The researchers found that no correlation could be made in either the West German or East German regions. Neither family, housing circumstances, working or leisure opportunities connected recognizably with the political orientations of those interviewed. Similarly, young people's dissatisfaction with their own life chances did not indicate any connections. Apparently an approval or rejection of right-wing orientations cannot be deduced from either socio-economic circumstances or subjective dissatisfactions (see also Held et al. 1991: 14).

Interestingly, typical patterns of justification seem to emerge in both East and West Germany. In East Germany, right-wing views are often connected with citizens' own discrimination. Belonging to the new Germany has led to discrimination towards non-German groups and it is clear that among the East German respondents there was a distinct connection between the agreement with nationalist orientations and a desire to be dissociated from socially lower persons (Held et al. 1995b: 33). In West Germany, however, the maintenance of living standards is validated by the assertion that one's own wealth and privileged status in the world is "self-earned" and in a certain way "results from the German nature". This therefore has to be defended against newcomers in the form of welfare chauvinism (Leiprecht 1991; Habermas 1993; Wahl 1993). These different patterns of excluding outsiders are connected to collective patterns of interpretations and ways of thinking in both East and West (Leiprecht 1993).

Is it the fault of single mothers and of anti-authoritarian education?

In West Germany the interest of young people in right-wing ideologies is usually interpreted as a result of societal processes of modernization and individualization. According to this view local communities, social groups, families and neighbourhoods are eroding. Consequently young people cannot fall back on traditional securities. The view is that the social processes of disintegration are leading to increasing orientational problems. In turn right-wing thinking becomes particularly attractive (Heitmeyer 1987, Heitmeyer et al. 1992). Although similar modernization and individualization has occurred in many societies it has not led to the violent racism evident in Germany. This view cannot therefore explain the specific political development of a country

(Leiprecht & Huber 1995). Interestingly, this explanation seems to fit with different political views. For example, in the Federal Republic of Germany, conservatives emphasize that violent young people lack security and conclude that neighbourhood and youth clubs can provide traditional values and act as a buffer against extreme right-wing young people. The conservative family policy also argues that women should be highly regarded for their role as mothers and believes that single mothers, high divorce rates, the emancipation of women, and the changing role of women and men leads to young people turning to right-wing activity.

The discourse emphasizing the central responsibilities of the family was also supported by left-wing social scientists. Under the heading "Education and the family has failed" the well-known sociologist Claus Leggewie, previously a member of the 1968 student movement, argues:

> The Nazi young people are branded as violent criminals in suspicious haste . . . Nobody has really shown them limits and offered themselves as role models: neither their parents, relatives, nor neighbours, friends, teachers, instructors or superiors! Let us listen to the sons and daughters. They demand authority, they have had enough of the non-seriousness of their elders (Leggewie 1993).

It is possible to find parents and teachers from the so-called 1968 generation who have created education in the style of "left fundamentalism". While there are many cases in which young people are moving to the right in order to oppose the left moralistic norm set by their parents and teachers, it does not make sense to deduce a general explanation in the way Leggewie has.

Although Leggewie's thesis is popular, research fails to support such a view. Analysis shows that young criminals come from all sorts of homes and families (Willems et al. 1993: 108). In fact, evidence indicates that young criminals are more likely to come from authoritarian families than from liberal homes (Utzmann-

Krombholz 1994) and the thesis of a "rebellion from the right" against anti-authoritarian parents cannot be substantiated. In the previously mentioned Tübingen study of young people in West and East Germany, 80 per cent of respondents who had nationalistic and racist views answered that their political opinions were similar to those of their parents. There is also a significant relationship between conventionalism and nationalist orientations (Held et al. 1995b: 14).

The acceptance by young people of dominant views and conventional attitudes can serve as an entry ticket into the social sphere and as a way of integrating themselves into society.

> When in crisis situations, stronger efforts at integration become necessary, and the dominant view of society, the state, political parties and the media supports tendencies of exclusion with nationalistic overtones. Conventionally oriented youth not only reproduce this, but drive it to the extreme. In this sense, right-wing extremism cannot be understood as a rebellion against the adult generation, or against the institutions of society, but rather as a sharpening of dominant views and tendencies (Held et al. 1995a: 124).

Gender and racism

Statistics in Germany indicate that 90 per cent of criminal racial offences and violent crimes are committed by men (Willems et al. 1993: 18; Utzmann-Krombholz 1994: 6). Empirical studies of young people provide a similar picture. Physical violence towards "foreigners" is therefore related to male young people (Riegel & Horn-Metzger 1995: 212). The difference between sexes is also found in voting patterns which indicate that two thirds of those voting for extreme right-wing parties are men and one third women. The study by Ursula Birsel shows that 15 per cent of young women and 36 per cent of young men supported extreme right-wing parties (Birsel 1993: 13). It would be wrong to conclude that these results have led to more research on the connection between male gender and racism, and an increase in new concepts in anti-racist work with young people. In fact, youth work practice and youth research has paid little attention to this worrying feature.

Research on racism has, however, been undertaken in the area of women's studies. Feminist researchers have critically asked why and how women become racist. While there is a much stronger tendency among male youth towards racist violence *on average*, this does not mean that young females are against violent or other forms of racism *in principle*. Male and female forms of racism thus have to be differentiated.

Contrary to earlier assumptions, the image of femininity propagated by right-wing extremist parties is not successful with young women (Oltmanns 1990; Holzkamp & Rommelspacher 1991; Siller 1991). Biologistic images are generally not accepted. Work and family planning are central emancipatory issues for young women, independent of whether they situate themselves on the "left" or on the "right" (Riegel & Horn-Metzger 1995: 211; Birsel & Busche-Baumann 1993: 27). The image of femininity of right-wing extremist parties seems to be more popular with male youth (Karl 1993: 41).

Returning to our consideration of males and females it is helpful to distinguish between direct personal physical violence towards "foreigners", and structural violence which is condoned by discrimination, exclusion and unequal treatment. Riegel & Horn-Metzger (1995) found that while the difference in behaviour between male and female young people is very clear in regard to personal violence, it is much less clear in relation to structural violence. This seems to support the thesis of Hilke Oltmanns that young females accept violence in a specific female form (Oltmanns 1990: 42).

Other attempts at an explanation emphasize the space occupied by males and females. Social "spaces – like streets, stadiums, squares, stations, pedestrian precincts during the day and night – are places which are frequented in different ways by women and girls, and by men" (Wobbe 1993: 110). It therefore seems to be obvious that racial violence by young males and men is linked to their occupation of these "public" social places.

Rommelspacher explains that young males' interest in right-wing activities is linked to how in our society we learn in early childhood to cope with the "strange" and the "other". The difference between the sexes when first engaging with other human beings is of fundamental importance. Socialization teaches boys to prove their masculinity by being aggressive and self-assertive, and by devaluing the feminine. Girls, on the other hand, develop their femininity in the form of peacefulness, caring and self-devaluation. Both are learning to cope with hierarchy and their place within it through domination or subordination (Rommelspacher 1992: 87). Both sexes seem to develop in different ways in regard to the "foreign" and the "other". This is connected to their position within hierarchies and leads to particular forms of racism and practices of exclusion. Those who are the subject of domination can in turn dominate the weak.

The approach Räthzel (1993) takes is helpful here. She asks whether women try to secure their position in existing gender relations by opposing refugees and immigrants. In this way women are participating in male-dominated structures.

Practical approaches in work with young people against racism and exclusion

Tackling racism and exclusion starts on different levels. There is, for example, action at the structural political level such as changing the law and providing equality with the right to vote. There is also a need to intervene where meanings are reproduced and communicated, such as in the media and in school. Similarly

111

there is a need to support groups that are targets of racism and help bring them to a "position of power". Finally, there is a need to create working approaches in different social-pedagogic fields and with different target groups.

There are now numerous examples of working approaches and practical proposals in the youth work literature. They range from anti-fascist and anti-racist actions and campaigns in the tradition of political movements, to different pedagogical approaches, to international youth meetings, intercultural youth work, local history projects, street work including mobile youth work and group work, and focused work with football fans (Hafemann 1989; Rajewski & Schmitz 1992; Posselt & Schumacher 1993). The discussion as to which approach is the best is inappropriate. There have to be different approaches for different contexts and for different target groups. The literature often indicates, however, that the same approaches can be used for all occasions and with all target groups.

Recently a discussion about so-called "acceptance youth work" has developed. This term was introduced by the Bremen-based social scientist Krafeld who argues that neither education nor punishment is really effective with right-wing young groups. Instead, he argues, young people's problems should be accepted (Krafeld et al. 1993: 92). This is a well-established educational principle of starting from the learner's position. However, the term is unsuitable here as it suggests that the young person's extreme right-wing views and racist behaviour should be accepted. In a public context which tends increasingly to accept the right, and which is dominated by a "discourse of the national", this term is inappropriate.

This view has led to the attempts by organized right-wing extremists to undertake their own political youth work (Ness 1993: 49). Academics such as Thomas Gehrmann of the Frankfurt Institut für Sozialarbeit und Sozial Pädagogik have proposed that acceptance youth work with right-wing youth groups should be supervised by right-wing social workers in order "to stabilise and not to destabilise the youth groups". Gehrmann hopes that working with such "stabilised groups" in accepted social spaces "off the streets" would lead to more satisfied young people who were less inclined to engage in violence (Mücke & Korn 1993: 110).

Krafeld and his co-workers have dissociated themselves from such models. For them the focus of the dispute and how change can take place is important. Their view is that social workers and young people are very different, and usually have contrary values and ways of understanding the world. The interpersonal communication between the workers and young people provides ways of listening to, and understanding, each other and to taking each other seriously (Krafeld 1993: 313). The prerequisite for the development of such processes is the hope that it will lead to change. For example, the offer of social rooms and practical support to assist young people to cope with problems all assists the process of communication and therefore understanding between practitioners and young people.

Developments have been made in intercultural work which has been used in multicultural neighbourhoods where there are "mixed" compositions of school classes, youth groups, kindergartens, urban quarters and so on. As a rule such concepts assume an encounter and meeting of different cultures in the hope that they will reduce prejudices (Schäfer & Six 1978; Hohmann & Reich 1989). In reality, however, it has become obvious that the best encounters are those where there is a degree of national or cultural homogenity (Akkent 1992: 153). The interest is in the "strange" and the "other" of immigrant culture and attitudes, and not the conditions of life (Kalpaka 1992: 136). Moreover, information about cultural differences of immigrant groups can scarcely reduce the negative views and evaluations made by Germans of non-Germans (see also, Lutz 1992).

Kalpaka argues that if we are really to combat racism there is a need to consider whether we should examine how "others" are presented. At the moment the "other" has negative implications (Kalpaka 1992: 136ff). She argues instead for models in which the "strange" is not used, preferring instead to see projects which attempt to help people to ask questions about their own society.

The question should not be what problems migrant children have, and if and when they want to return to their home countries, but rather what problems are the schools imposing on young people, and what must be changed in the host society in order for them to enjoy living in Germany. In this way the main focus is shifted from the "other" to the host society (Kalpaka 1992: 140).

Conclusion

In conclusion, we would like to make some central points. When we are working as professionals with young people we are not exclusively teachers or youth workers. We are also in a broad sense members of society. We have a certain share in the responsibility for developments in society as well as in the school or in the youth centre. Teachers should not exclusively limit their roles to what is generally understood as real pedagogy (for example the teaching of knowledge in the classroom, the counselling conversation by a youth worker in the youth centre, etc.). It is in the broad sense that there are real possibilities to act. With critical reflection teachers and youth workers cannot ignore the structures that dominate the pedagogical relationship.

In anti-racist youth work racism is often described as something "bad" or "evil": young people therefore need to be educated. This concept is supported by the thesis that these young people do not know any different because they are less intelligent or are stupid. In such a view the teacher seems to be "above everybody", "intelligent", "good" and "free from racism" and the young people are "inferior", "stupid", "bad", "with deficiencies" and "are evil".

It seems to us more reasonable not to understand racism or anti-racism as something which is planted in a certain way as a definite factor in the single human being. Rather it is more helpful to consider both racism and anti-racism as ways of thinking and actions which relate to specific situations. On the one hand we have to search for something "evil" in our human being. On the other hand it is clear that as teachers and youth workers we can offer situations and alternatives of action for the young people with whom we are working.

Notes

1. In 1989, 121,000 people applied for political asylum in Germany, in 1991, 256,000 applied and in 1992, 438,000 (Mühlhum 1993). In recent years, most of the applicants have come from war zones in what was previously Yugoslavia and from Romania. In 1989 a further 377,036 people from Romania, Poland and the former Soviet Union immigrated as *Aussiedler* and in 1992, 230,000 (Ronge 1993).
2. Remarkably enough, a further group was completely ignored in the numbers game as played by many politicians. Namely, the additional 230,000 workers who travelled annually to Germany as employees of German businesses: they worked as seasonal and contract workers with temporary work permits (Ronge 1993: 21).
3. This can also be confirmed by a glance at the *Handbuch der Jugendforschung* (Handbook of Youth Research) (Krüger 1992).

References and further reading

Akkent, M. 1992. Praktische Möglichkeiten zur Bearbeitung kulturzentristischer Denk- und Handlungsmuster in der Arbeit mit Jugendlichen. See Leiprecht (ed.) 1992, 153–69.
Autrata, O., G. Kaschuba, R. Leiprecht & C. Wolf (eds) 1989. *Theorien über Rassismus*. Berlin/Hamburg: Argument.
Bade, K. J. (ed.) 1985. *Auswanderer – Wanderarbeiter – Gastarbeiter. Bevölkerung, Arbeitsmarkt und Wanderungen in Deutschland seit der Mitte des 19. Jahrhunderts*. Ostfildern: Harald Winkel.
Bade, K. J. (ed.) 1993. *Deutsche im Ausland – Fremde in Deutschland. Migration in Geschichte und Gegenwart*. München: Beck.
Birsel, U. 1993. Mädchen und Rechtsextremismus. Rechtsextrem-

istische Orientierungen bei weiblichen und männlichen Jugendlichen. *Jugendpolitik*, **3**, 12–14.

Birsel, U. & M. Busche-Baumann 1993. Gewerkschaftliche Strategien gegen rechtsextremistische Orientierungen bei Auszubildenden. *Die Mitbestimmung. Monatszeitschrift der Hans-Böckler-Stiftung* **4**, 27–30.

Brozinsky-Schwabe, E. 1990. Die DDR-Bürger im Umgang mit "Fremden". See S. Kleff, E. Brozinsky-Schwabe, M-T. Albert, H. Marburger & M-E. Karsten 1990, 18–44.

Brück, W. 1988. *Das "Skinhead"-Phänomen aus jugendkriminologischer Sicht, Expertise des Zentralinstituts für Jugendforschung.* Leipzig: Zentralinstitut für Jugendforschung.

Bundes-Kriminalamt 1995. *Datenmaterial aus der Kriminalstatistik zu fremdenfeindlich motivierten Straf- und Gewalttaten.* Meckenheim: Bundes-Kriminalamt.

Castels, S. 1987. *Migration und Rassismus in Westeuropa.* Berlin: Express.

DJI – Deutsches Jugendinstitut 1993. *Gewalt gegen Fremde. Rechtsradikale, Skinheads und Mitläufer.* München: Verlag Deutsches Jugendinstitut (DJI).

Engelmann, B. 1984. *Du deutsch? Geschichte der Ausländer in unserem Land.* München: Bertelsmann.

Foitzik, A., R. Leiprecht, A. Marvakis & U. Seid (eds) 1992. *Ein Herrenvolk von Untertanen. Rassismus – Nationalismus – Sexismus.* Duisburg: DISS.

Ford, G. (Berichterstatter) 1990. Europäisches Parlament, Bericht des Untersuchungsausschußes zu Rassismus und Ausländerfeindlichkeit in der Europäischen Gemeinschaft vom 23.Juli 1990.

Gerhard, U. 1991. *"Wenn Flüchtlinge und Einwanderer zu 'Asylantenfluten' werden ..." – Eine kommentierte Dokumentation zum Rassismus im Mediendiskurs.* Bochum: Diskurswerkstatt.

Gillmeister, H. & H. Kurthen 1989. *Ausländerbeschäftigung in der Krise? Die Beschäftigungschancen ausländischer Arbeitnehmer am Beispiel der West-Berliner Industrie.* Berlin: Rainer Bohn.

Granato, M. 1995. Jugend in Europa. Ausbildung und Berufseinstieg von Jugendlichen aus Migrantenfamilien. *BWP – Berufsbildung in Wissenschaft und Praxis – Zeitschrift des Bundesinstituts für Berufsbildung,* **2**, 10–14.

Habermas, J. 1993. *Vergangenheit als Zukunft. Das alte Deutschland im neuen Europa?* München: Piper.

Hafemann, H. 1989. Ansätze und Probleme einer Jugendarbeit mit rechtsextrem orientierten Jugendlichen. *Jugendschutz*, **6**, 12–22.

Heil, H., M. Perik & P-U. Wendt (eds) 1993. *Jugend und Gewalt. Über den Umgang mit gewaltbereiten Jugendlichen.* Marburg: Schüren (SP).

Heinemann, K-H. & Schubarth, W. (eds) 1992. *Der antifaschistische Staat entläßt seine Kinder. Jugend und Rechtsextremismus in Ostdeutschland.* Köln: Pappyrossa.

Heitmeyer, W. 1987. *Rechtsextremistische Orientierungen bei Jugendlichen – Empirische Ergebnisse und Erklärungsmuster einer Untersuchung zur politischen Sozialisation.* Weinheim-München: Juventa.

Heitmeyer, W. et al. 1992. *Die Bielefelder Rechtsextremismus-Studie – Erste Langzeituntersuchung zur politischen Sozialisation männlicher Jugendlicher.* Weinheim-München: Juventa.

Held, J., H. Horn, R. Leiprecht & A. Marvakis 1991. "Du mußt so handeln, daß Du Gewinn machst und theoretische Uberlegungen zu Politischen" *Empirische Untersuchungen Orientierungen bei jugendlichen Arbeitnehmerinnen.* Duisburg: DISS.

Held, J., H-W. Horn & A. Marvakis 1995a. See Leiprecht 1995, 111–132.

Held, J., H-W. Horn & A. Marvakis 1995b. Gespaltene Jugend. *Politische Orientierungen jugendlicher ArbeitnehmerInnen und ihre subjektiven Begründungen im Kontext gesellschaftlicher Veränderungen.* Research report. Düsseldorf: Hans-Böckler-Stiftung.

Herbert, U. 1986. *Geschichte der Ausländerbeschäftigung in Deutschland von 1880 bis 1980: Saisonarbeiter – Zwangsarbeiter – Gastarbeiter.* Berlin/Bonn: J. H. W. Dietz Nachf.

Hobsbawm, E. J. 1991. *Nationen und Nationalismus. Mythos und Realität seit 1780.* Frankfurt a.M.: Campus.

Hohmann, M. & H. H. Reich (eds) 1989. *Ein Europa für Mehrheiten und Minderheiten. Diskussion um interkulturelle Erziehung.* Münster/New York: Waxmann.

Holzkamp, C. & B. Rommelspacher 1991. Frauen und Rechtsextremismus. *Päd.Extra/Demokratische Erziehung*, 1, 33–9.

Huhnke, B. 1993. Intermediale Abhängigkeiten bei der Inszenierung rassistischer Feindbilder seit Mitte der achtziger Jahre am Beispiel der Wochenzeitungen *Bild am Sonntag* und *Der Spiegel.* See Jäger & Link 1993, 213–66.

Institut zur sozialpädagogischen Forschung Mainz (ISM) e.V. 1993. *Rassismus – Fremdenfeindlichkeit – Rechtsextremismus: Beiträge zu einem gesellschaftlichen Diskurs.* Bielefeld: KT-Verlag.

Inowlocki, L. 1992. Zum Mitgliedschaftsprozeß Jugendlicher in rechtsextremen Gruppen. *Psychosozial 51*, 15(III), 54–6.

Inowlocki, L. 1996. *Geschichtsbezüge im Mitgliedschaftssprozeß Jugendlicher in rechtsextremen Gruppen.* Weinheim: Deutscher Studien Verlag.

Jäger, S. & J. Link (eds) 1993. *Die vierte Gewalt – Rassismus und die Medien,* Duisburg: DISS.

Jäger, S., H. Kellershohn & J. Pfenning (eds) 1993. *SchlagZeilen –*

Rostock: Rassismus in den Medien. Duisburg: DISS.

Kalpaka, A. 1992. Überlegungen zur antirassistischen Praxis mit Jugendlichen in der BRD. See Leiprecht (ed.) 1992, 131–52.

Kalpaka, A. & N. Räthzel (eds) 1990. *Die Schwierigkeit, nicht rassistisch zu sein*. Leer: Mundo.

Karl, H. 1993. Auf der Suche nach dem rechten Mann – Jungen auf dem Weg zur Männlichkeit. *Offene Jugendarbeit – Zeitschrift für Jugendhäuser, Jugendzentren, Spielmobile*. Stuttgart **4**, 37–42.

Katsoulis, H. 1984. *Bürger zweiter Klasse. Ausländer in der Bundesrepublik*. Berlin: Express.

Kleff, S., E. Brozinsky-Schwabe, M-T. Albert, H. Marburger & M-E. Karsten (eds) 1990. *BRD – DDR – Alte und neue Rassismen im Zuge der deutsch-deutschen Einigung*. Frankfurt a.M.: Verlag für Interkulturelle Kommunikation (IKO).

Klönne, A. 1987. Die deutsche Geschichte geht weiter. *Das Argument* **161**. Hamburg-Berlin: Auschwitz ins Museum.

Krafeld, F. J. 1993. Jugendarbeit mit rechten Jugendszenen. Konzeptionelle Grundlagen und praktische Erfahrungen. See Otto & Merten 1993, 310–24.

Krafeld, F. J., E. Lutzebäck, G. Scharr, C. Storm & W. Welp 1993. Akzeptierende Jugendarbeit mit rechtsextremen Jugendlichen? Konzeptionelle Grundlinien praktischer Erfahrungen. See Heil et al. 1993, 91–100.

Krüger, H.-H. 1992. *Handbuch der Jugendforschung*. Opladen: Leske & Budrich.

Kühne, P. 1987. Die Trennungslinien werden schärfer – Ausländische Arbeitnehmer in den Gewerkschaften. *Monatszeitung Expreß*, **6**.

Kühnl, R. (ed.) 1974. *Texte zur Faschismusdiskussion. Positionen und Kontroversen*. Reinbek bei Hamburg: Rowohlt.

Langer, H. 1991. Rechtsextremismus von Jugendlichen in der DDR. *1999, Zeitschrift für Sozialgeschichte des 20. und 21. Jahrhunderts*, **1**. 89–99.

Leggewie, C. 1993. Education in the family has failed. *Die Zeit*. **3**, vol. 14, No. 1–2.

Leiprecht, R. 1990. *"Da baut sich ja in uns ein Haß auf" Zur subjektiven Funktionalität von Rassismus und Ethnozentrismus bei abhängig beschäftigten Jugendlichen*. Hamburg/Berlin: Argument.

Leiprecht, R. 1991. *"Rassismus und Ethnozentrismus – Zu den unterschiedlichen Formen dieser ausgrenzenden und diskriminierenden Orientierungen und Praxen und zur Notwendigkeit einer mehrdimensionalen antirassistischen Praxis"*. Duisburg: DISS.

Leiprecht, R. (ed.) 1992. *Unter Anderen – Rassismus und Jugendarbeit*. Duisburg: DISS.

Leiprecht, R. 1992. Ein Problem nur für "Fremde"? Rassismus – die Macht der Zuschreibung. *Widersprüche,* **43**(12), 17–34.

Leiprecht, R. 1993. Das Modell "unmittelbare" und/oder "direkte Konkurrenz": Erklärung oder Rechtfertigung von Rechtsextremismus. See Institut zur sozialpädagogischen Forschung Mainz (ISM) e.V. 1993, 68–86.

Leiprecht, R. (ed.) 1995. "In Grenzen Verstickt". Jugenliche und Rassismus in Europa. Duisburg: DISS.

Leiprecht, R. & C. Huber 1995. "Nationale" Orientierungen bei deutschen und niederländischen Jugendlichen. See Leiprecht (ed.) 1995, 56–90.

Loose, I. 1993. "Eine feste Burg" – Wie eine süddeutsche Zeitung das Hohelied von der "Festung Europa" singt. Duisburg: DISS.

Lutz, H. 1992. Ist Kultur Schicksal? Über die gesellschaftliche Konstruktion von Kultur und Migration. See Leiprecht 1992, 43–62.

Meulemann, H. & A. Elting-Camus (eds) 1993. *Deutscher Soziologentag. Lebensverhältnisse und soziale Konflikte im neuen Europa.* Opladen: Westdeutscher Verlag.

Meyer, A. & K-K. Rabe 1979. *Unsere Stunde die wird kommen – Rechtsextremismus unter Jugendlichen.* Bornheim-Merten: Lamuv.

Miles, R. 1989. Bedeutungskonstitution und der Begriff des Rassismus. *Das Argument,* **175**, 5/6, 353–68.

Miles, R. 1991. *Rassismus – Einführung in die Geschichte und Theorie eines Begriffs,* Hamburg: Argument.

Mücke, T. & J. Korn 1993. Miteinander statt Gegeneinander. Neue Wege in der Jugendarbeit – Dialogversuch mit rechtsextrem orientierten Jugendlichen. See Heil et al. 1993, 146–57.

Mühlhum, A. 1993. Armutswanderung, Asyl und Abwehrverhalten. Globale und nationale Dilemmata. In *Aus Politik und Zeitgeschichte. Beilage zur Wochenzeitung Das Parlament.* B7/93 vom 12.Februar 1993. 3–15.

Ness, K. 1993. Alles nur "Einzeltäter und verwirrte Jugendliche"? See Heil et al. 1993, 39–52.

Oltmanns, H. 1990. Siegen, kämpfen, durchgreifen lassen. Rechtsextremismus bei Mädchen. *Widersprüche* **35**(6), 41–5.

Osterkamp, U. 1989. Gesellschaftliche Widersprüche und Rassismus. See Autrata, O., G. Kaschuba, R. Leiprecht & C. Wolf 1989, 113–34.

Otto, H-U. & R. Merten (eds) 1993. *Rechtsradikale Gewalt im vereinigten Deutschland. Jugend im gesellschaftlichen Umbruch.* Bonn: Bundeszentrale für poltische Bildung.

Page Moch, L. 1992. *Moving Europeans. Migration in Western Europe since 1650.* Bloomington, Indiana: University Press.

Paul, G. & B. Schoßig (eds) 1979. *Jugend und Neofaschismus – Provokation oder Identifikation?* Frankfurt a.M.: Europäische Verlagsanstalt (EVA).

Posselt, R. E. & K. Schumacher 1993. *Projekthandbuch: Gewalt und Rassismus.* Mülheim a.d.R.: Verlag an der Ruhr.

Quinkert, A. & S. Jäger 1991. *Warum dieser Haß in Hoyerswerda? Die rassistische Hetze von Bild gegen Flüchtlinge im Herbst 1991.* Duisburg: DISS.

Rajewski, C. & A. Schmitz 1992. *Wegzeichen – Initiativen gegen Rechtsextremismus und Ausländerfeindlichkeit.* Tübingen: Verein für Friedenspädagogik.

Räthzel, N. 1993. Selbstunterwerfung in Bildern der Anderen. See WIDEE 1993, 145–75.

Räthzel, N. & Ü. Sarica 1994. *Migration und Diskriminierung in der Arbeit: Das Beispiel Hamburg.* Hamburg: Argument.

Riegel, C. & T. Horn-Metzger 1995. Geschlecht und politische Orientierungen. Zur Notwendigkeit einer geschlechtsspezifischen Herangehensweise. See Held et al. 1995b, 207–36.

Rommelspacher, B. 1992. Rechtsextremismus und Dominanzkultur. In Foitzik, A. & R. Leiprecht, A. Marvakis & U. Seid 1992, 81–94.

Rosenthal, G. 1992. Kollektives Schweigen zu den Nazi-Verbrechen. *Psychosozial 51,* 15.Jahrgang, 3. 22–33.

Ruhrmann, G. 1987. *Ausländerberichterstattung in der Kommune. Inhaltsanalyse Bielefelder Tageszeitungen unter Berücksichtigung "ausländerfeindlicher" Alltagstheorien.* Opladen: Leske & Budrich.

Schafer, B. & U. Six 1978. *Sozialpsychologie des Vozurtells.* Kohlhammer: Stuttgart/Berlin/Cologne/Mainz.

Schiebel, M. 1992. Biographische Selbstdarstellungen rechtsextremer und ehemals rechtsextremer Jugendlicher. *Psychosozial 51,* 15.Jahrgang, 3, 66–77.

Schubarth, W. 1993. Die Suche nach Gewißheit. Rechtsextremismus als Verarbeitungsform des gesellschaftlichen Umbruchs. See Otto & Merten 1993, 256–66.

Schubarth, W. & T. Schmidt 1992. "Sieger der Geschichte". Verordneter Antifaschismus und die Folgen. See Heinemann & Schubarth 1992, 12–28.

Seifert, W. 1992. *Ausländer in der Bundesrepublik – Soziale und ökonomische Mobilität.* Berlin: Wissenschaftszentrum Berlin für Sozialforschung.

Seifert, W. 1993. Ökonomische und soziale Mobilität von Ausländern in der Bundesrepublik Deutschland. In *Acta Demographica,* 1993. 79–92.

Siller, G. 1991. Junge Frauen und Rechtsextremismus – Zum Zusammenhang von weiblichen Lebenserfahrungen und rechtsextremistischem Gedankengut. *Deutsche Jugend*, 1, 23–32.

Statistisches Bundesamt 1995. Statistisches Jahrbuch 1994 für die Bundesrepublik Deutschland. Wiesbaden: Metzler-Poeschel.

Tränhardt, D., R. Dieregsweiler & B. Santel 1995. *Einwanderer in Nordrhein-Westfalen. Wissenschaftliches Gutachten zur Lebenssituation der Menschen aus den Anwerbeländern mit ausländischer Staatsangehörigkeit und zu den Handlungsprioritäten der Politik.* Research report Ministerium für Arbeit, Gesundheit und Soziales Nordrhein-Westfalen. Teil II.

Uihlein, H. & W. Weber 1989. *Denn wir sind Fremdlinge vor Dir – Werkheft Asyl*. Karlsruhe-Freiburg-Stuttgart: Caritas Verband für Württemberg e.V.

Utzmann-Krombholz, H. 1994. *Rechtsextremismus und Gewalt: Affinitäten und Resitenzen von Mädchen und jungen Frauen*. Research report. Düsseldorf: Ministerium für die Gleichstellung von Frau und Mann Nordrhein-Westfalen.

Wahl, K. 1993. Fremdenfeindlichkeit, Rechtsextremismus, Gewalt. Eine Synopse wissenschaftlicher Untersuchungen und Erklärungsansätze. See DJI 1993, 11–68.

Weiß, K. 1989. Die braune Stafette. *ZEIT-magazin*, 27.

WIDEE (eds) 1993. *Nahe Fremde – fremde Nähe*. Wien: Wiener Frauenverlag.

Willems, H. & S. Würtz, R. Eckert 1993. *Fremdenfeindliche Gewalt: Eine Analyse von Täterstrukturen und Eskalationsprozessen*. Research report. Bonn: Bundesministerium Familie und Jugend.

Wobbe, T. 1993. Geschlechterverteilung im sozialen Raum. See Meulemann & Elting-Camus 1993, 113–16.

6

Towards multi-cultural and anti-racist youth work in Flanders

Danny Wildemeersch and Gie Redig

Introduction

Racism in general, and among young people in particular, has become increasingly explicit in Flanders during recent years. The political expression of this racism has been a party called the Vlaams Blok (the Flemish Bloc). At the end of the 1970s the party was established by right-wing activists within the centrist nationalist party, the Volksunie (the People's Union). The leaders of the Vlaams Blok presented a much more radical and separatist programme in relation to Flemish nationalist aspirations than the Volksunie. In the course of the 1980s, however, the Vlaams Blok gradually reoriented its goals with Flemish nationalism being replaced by a racist focus on the migrant population in Flanders. The new party line was strongly inspired by the racist ideas of similar movements abroad, like the Front National of Le Pen in France. As a consequence, the party moved from a marginal position, rapidly gaining popularity. During the November 1991 parliamentary elections, the Vlaams Blok obtained some 12 per cent of the votes in the Flemish community securing one in four votes cast in the important Flemish city of Antwerp. This position was confirmed in the municipal elections of 1994.

The growing success of the Vlaams Blok alarmed many politicians in traditional parties as well as members of key social movements, leading to a number of different initiatives including the appointment of a Royal Commissioner for Migrants' Affairs. As is often the case in times of social or political crisis, youth and youth organizations were invited to take action. Together with schools, youth organizations were, and · increasingly still are, expected to influence the younger generation in respect of multiculturalism and challenge racism. Furthermore, youth organizations are expected to prepare their members for their future role in society. Today the responsibility of youth *vis-à-vis* society is increasing, both from a demographic and a socio-economic point of view: the Belgian population is ageing, while the relative number of young people within this population is decreasing. Yet the relative number of young people with a non-Belgian origin is growing with reference to the global youth population. For this reason, the quality of tomorrow's society will partly depend on the qualities of this category of youth (Anon 1992: 7).

In this chapter, we will describe the present expectations *vis-à-vis* youth and youth organizations in respect of racism and multiculturalism, and what initiatives have been taken to date. This discussion will be preceded by selected background information concerning the political situation in Belgium in general and Flanders in particular, including the presentation of research results relating to the attitude of Belgian/Flemish inhabitants towards foreigners.

Background information

Foreigners often have great difficulty in understanding the political scene in Belgium. It is indeed a complex one, as there are three official linguistic communities: the French-speaking (43 per cent); the Dutch speaking (56.8 per cent); and the German speaking (0.2 per cent) communities. There are also three distinct regions: the Walloon region; the Flemish region; and the Brussels region. This situation is the result of three major constitutional changes that have taken place since 1975. These changes, which have turned Belgium into a federal state, are the result of ethnic/linguistic/political conflicts among the French and Dutch-speaking communities, and have created problems in political, social and cultural life ever since the kingdom of Belgium was established in 1830.

The Flemish community has a population of some 5.7 million inhabitants in a total Belgian population of 10 million. Situated in the north of the country, the Flemish region was, until the Second World War, mainly an agrarian community, which explains its previously relatively weak position in the Belgium economic and political context. Since the 1950s, however, Flanders has rapidly industrialized and become the dominant centre of economic activity in the country. Whereas Wallonia derived its economic structure from the first industrial revolution in the nineteenth century, Flanders was economically restructured during the industrial revolution after the Second World War. This also explains why the Walloon region, the Flemish region and the Brussels region experienced a different influx of migrant workers during their recent history.

Belgium has been a multi-ethnic society ever since it came into existence with cultural diversity being one of its main characteristics. At the beginning of the twentieth century 212,474 foreigners lived in the country. This figure represents one quarter of the current foreign population. From the 1920s onwards, cultural and ethnic diversity increased, with workers particularly from Poland, the former Czechslovakia, Yugoslavia and Italy settling in Belgium. These migrant workers were attracted as cheap labour, especially into the mining industries. From 1946 to 1956 various contracts between the Belgian and the Italian states assisted the immigration of tens of thousands of southern Italian workers. These workers had to live and work in uncomfortable and unhealthy conditions and among the people who lost their lives in the disasters in the Belgian coal mines there was always a considerable number of Italians. From 1956 onwards a further diversification took place with a ban on Italian immigration. Belgium was then forced to search for cheap labour from elsewhere and began to attract workers from Spain, Greece, Morocco and Turkey. During the economic expansion of the 1960s there was a great need for unqualified labour in Belgium's larger urban centres. Hence, the Belgian embassies in the Magreb countries organized campaigns to persuade peasants to try their luck in this promising foreign country. This led to the high concentration of migrant populations in larger cities like Brussels, Antwerp, Liège and Gent, as well as in smaller towns like Mechelen, Ciloorde and St Niklaas.

During the 1960s and 1970s three major developments took place with respect to the influx of migrants in Belgium:
1. a rapid growth in the migrant population, both in absolute and in relative terms, from 453,500 (4.93 per cent of the total population) to 891,250 (9.04 per cent of the total population) in 1983.
2. a shift of the migrant population from industrial zones to urban centres which usually led to large concentrations of migrant families in materially poor inner city areas.
3. a complex situation of cohabitation with several generations of the same or different nationalities of migrants, including a large number of young people, living in confined areas of the old urban quarters. Here they lived close to a poor and ageing Belgian population.

In 1974 a formal stop to immigration was decreed marking the beginning of a slow process of integration of communities of migrant workers and ethnic minorities into Belgian society. Gradually many migrant families began to realize that their stay in the host country was to be permanent, leading them to search for more appropriate housing.

In order to complete the picture, we present tables which provide information on the presence of migrants in the different regions of Belgian society. It should be noted that with respect to the issue of immigration, figures are of relative importance.

Indeed, many "foreigners" have, over the years, taken the opportunity to become naturalized and hence have become Belgians.
Yet the ownership of a Belgian identity card is no defence against
discrimination and intolerance.

Table 6.1 The distribution of inhabitants of foreign nationality over
the three Belgian regions.

		Flanders	Wallonia	Brussels	Kingdom
1970	N	164,029	358,746	173,507	696,282
	% total	3.0	11.4	16.1	7.2
1981	N	232,544	408,158	237,875	878,577
	% total	4.1	12.7	23.9	8.9
1984	N	240,387	402,209	248,217	890,873
	% total	4.2	12.5	25.3	9.0
1985	N	243,405	401,967	252,258	897,630
	% total	4.3	12.5	25.7	9.1
1986	N	222,619	375,792	248,131	846,482
	% total	3.9	11.7	25.4	8.6
1987	N	226,145	374,333	252,269	853,247
	% total	4.0	11.7	25.9	8.6
1988	N	235,611	368,750	258,138	862,499
	% total	4.1	11.4	26.6	8.7
1989	N	238,117	366,618	264,022	868,757
	% total	4.2	11.2	27.2	8.8

Source: National Statistical Institute.

Table 6.1 indicates that in the Brussels region more than one
quarter of the population is composed of foreigners, whereas
Flanders has only some 4 per cent of inhabitants of foreign
nationality, and Wallonia 11 per cent. These figures have also
changed since the 1970s. Table 6.2 provides a clearer picture of
this.

Table 6.2 shows that the distribution of the foreign population
in general over the three Belgian regions has changed since 1970.
Flanders has slightly, and Brussels more markedly, increased its
share in foreign populations, whereas the Walloon region has
slightly decreased its share. As far as Brussels is concerned, it
must be remembered that the city has played an increasingly
important role in the EU political scene, which explains the

Table 6.2 The evolution of the relative presence of foreigners per region.

	Flanders	Wallonia	Brussels	Belgium
1970	23.6	51.5	24.9	100.0
1981	26.5	46.5	27.0	100.0
1984	27.0	45.2	28.0	100.0
1985	27.1	44.8	28.1	100.0
1986	26.3	44.4	29.3	100.0
1987	26.5	43.9	29.6	100.0
1988	27.3	42.7	29.9	100.0
1989	27.4	42.2	30.4	100.0

Source: National Statistical Institute.

Table 6.3 The foreigners per nationality and their distribution.

Nationality	Total	%	Flanders (%)	Wallonia (%)	Brussels (%)
Italian	241,006	27.7	10.8	75.7	13.5
Moroccan	135,464	15.6	29.1	15.5	55.4
French	91,444	10.5	15.5	56.3	28.1
Turkish	79,460	9.1	49.5	25.4	25.1
Dutch	60,533	7.0	83.0	9.7	7.3
Spanish	52,549	6.0	18.0	31.7	50.3
German	26,405	3.0	36.4	46.2	17.5
British	21,805	2.5	49.0	21.6	29.4
Greek	20,613	2.4	17.0	31.2	51.8
Portugese	13,498	1.6	16.4	25.5	58.1
American (US)	11,624	1.3	31.0	48.1	20.9
Zairian	10,871	1.3	12.6	34.0	53.4
Algerian	10,647	1.2	13.8	62.5	23.7
Tunisian	6,244	0.7	32.8	20.3	46.9
Yugoslavian	5,350	0.6	20.5	30.3	49.2
Luxemburgian	4,771	0.5	14.6	50.1	35.4
Polish	4,709	0.5	23.5	60.7	15.8
Others	71,764	8.3	30.6	25.4	44.0
Total	868,757	100.0	27.4	42.2	30.3

Source: National Statistic Institute and figures provided by the National Register.

presence of a number of EU foreigners. More detailed information about the type of nationality with respect to the various regions is given in Table 6.3.

Table 6.3 provides us with a more detailed picture of the distribution of the various nationalities over the three regions. We will restrict our comments to the major groups of migrant labourers. The Italians still represent the majority of foreigners and are mainly concentrated in Wallonia, due primarily to their former employment in the mining industries. The majority of Moroccans live in Brussels, while there are also a large number of them living in Flanders. Almost half of the Turkish population live in Flanders, whereas Wallonia and Brussels each have about one quarter of the Turkish population that lives in Beligium.

Young people in Belgian and Flemish society

Before discussing the role of youth work and youth organizations in relation to multiculturalism and anti-racism, it is important to provide background data on young people in general, and of migrant youth in particular, in Belgian and Flemish society. When we speak about "youth" in this context, we refer to the age group of 0–25 years, although we know that in the Anglo-Saxon tradition the category "youth" usually means 15–25 years. In Belgium, there were 3,189,338 young people as at 1 January 1991, among whom 11.10 per cent were of non-Belgian nationality (5.27 per cent EU and 5.83 per cent non-EU). Flanders has a population of 1,831,006 young people, or 31.75 per cent of the total Flemish population, among whom 5.84 per cent has a non-Belgian nationality (2.17 per cent EU and 3.67 per cent non-EU). In Brussels, however, the situation is entirely different. Brussels has 291,804 young people, representing 30.39 per cent of the total Brussels population. Almost four in ten young inhabitants living in Brussels are of non-Belgian nationality (39.2 per cent) of whom 13.47 per cent are of EU nationality and 26.45 per cent have a non-EU nationality.

Focusing on migrant young people in Flanders, we need to record that this population is both heterogeneous and dynamic. Some of the migrant young people are able to benefit from Belgian society, whereas others are seriously at risk of margin-

Table 6.4 Youth with foreign nationalities in Flanders.

	0–14	%	15–24	%	<25 yr	%	≥25 yr	%	General total	% compared to foreigners
Total neighbouring countries	8,830	11.03	11,442	14.29	20,272	25.32	59,791	74.68	80,063	32.08
Greece	637	16.67	623	16.30	1,260	32.98	2,561	67.02	3,821	1.48
Spain	1,520	15.64	1,663	17.11	3,183	32.75	6,535	67.25	9,718	3.77
Portugal	435	16.97	407	15.84	843	32.81	1,726	67.19	2,569	1.00
Italy	5,076	18.82	4,589	17.02	9,665	35.84	17,501	64.16	26,966	10.47
Total Mediterranean	7,669	17.80	7,282	16.91	14,951	34.71	28,123	65.29	43,074	16.72
Total other EU	2,793	20.81	1,800	13.41	4,593	34.21	8,831	65.79	13,424	5.21
Total EU	19,292	14.14	20,524	15.04	39,816	29.18	96,745	70.89	136,467	52.97
Total other European countries	1,111	15.73	937	13.26	2,048	28.99	5,017	71.01	7,065	2.74
Turkey	17,837	42.13	8,684	20.51	26,521	62.64	15,818	37.36	42,339	16.43
Algeria	450	29.11	206	13.32	656	42.43	890	57.57	1,546	0.60
Morocco	19,385	45.70	8,133	19.17	27,518	64.87	14,900	35.13	42,418	16.46
Tunisia	779	36.92	272	12.89	1,051	49.81	1,059	50.19	2,110	0.82
Other nationalities	5,487	21.35	3,981	15.49	8,468	36.85	16,228	63.15	25,696	9.97
Total foreigners	64,341	24.97	42,737	16.59	107,078	41.56	150,657	54.48	257,641	100.0
Belgians	971,725	17.64	752,203	13.65	1,723,928	31.29	3,785,912	68.71	5,509,840	100.0
Total population	1,036,306	17.96	794,940	13.78	1,831,006	31.75	3,936,569	68.25	5,767,575	100.0

Source: National Statistic Institute, 1991.

alization. The group that suffers most from poverty come from non-EU countries such as Turkey, Algeria, Morocco and Tunisia, and to a lesser extent those from Mediterranean EU countries like Greece, Spain, Portugal and Italy. Table 6.4 shows numbers and percentages of these categories in Flanders.

Racism and anti-racist policy in Belgium and Flanders

As referred to in the introduction, racism *vis-à-vis* the migrant population has become increasingly explicit since the 1980s, entering the political scene, especially in Flanders, via the emergence of the Vlaams Blok. This political party contains a variety of feelings of discontent, while mainly focusing on the presence of migrants in Flemish society. Hence, these election results suggest that racist feelings are stronger in Flanders than in Brussels and Wallonia, although as we have seen the presence of migrants is much more prominent in the latter regions. To date there are few satisfactory explanations for these registered differences in voting behaviour among the regions. Furthermore, these differences in voting patterns contradict some of the research findings relating to the attitudes towards foreigners in the three Belgian regions.

Billiet et al. (1990), who conducted several empirical research projects on racism, found that the negative feelings towards foreign groups are stronger in Wallonia than in Flanders, whereas the Brussels region occupies a "middle position". Hence, Flanders seems to have the most tolerant attitude towards foreigners. While trying to find an explanation for this phenomenon, researchers related the negative attitude towards foreigners to a more global attitude of ethnocentrism. Ethnocentrism means that one group considers other groups as inferior, believing their own ethnic group to be superior. The research shows that the Flemish have a fairly positive attitude towards themselves,

131

whereas the Walloons have a relatively negative self-identity. Again, the inhabitants of the Brussels region occupy a "middle position". According to the authors this positive self-attitude of the Flemish is the result of a long-lasting historical process of emancipation. Furthermore, at the time of writing, the socio-economic situation in this region is relatively good. Finally, the Flemish have had few contacts with foreigners in their daily life. According to the researchers, the combination of these factors explains the fairly tolerant attitude of the Flemish.

The research demonstrates that the inhabitants of the Walloon region are more negative in their judgement of foreigners. The authors ascribe these negative feelings to a fairly negative self-image, combined with less prosperous socio-economic conditions, and a sustained presence of foreigners. Whereas Wallonia has more characteristics of a multi-cultural society than Flanders, its population was observed to have a more negative attitude towards foreigners living in materially poorer conditions. In Wallonia the competition with migrants, both in the labour market and with respect to welfare services, is fiercer than in Flanders. In other words, it is easier to be more tolerant in Flanders as there are far fewer migrants present in society, and because the positive economic situation prevents the migrants from being experienced as competitors.

The researchers also investigated some of the basic mechanisms of intolerance, finding age to be an important variable. The higher the age, the higher the rate of intolerance towards foreigners. They also found that racial intolerance is characteristic of people who have had a problematic school career. People who have finished grammar school are much more tolerant than people who have acquired a vocational or technical degree. Furthermore, the level of income is an important variable. The higher the income, the higher the tolerance towards foreigners. Similarly, the lower the income, the lower the racial tolerance. Finally, the degree of social integration plays an important role. The better one is integrated, the more one is tolerant towards foreigners. People who lack social contacts, or who are badly integrated in normative social networks, tend to be unsympathetic towards foreigners.

The same research has further considered attitudes of Flemish young adults towards migrant workers. The examination by Waege (1991) of a representative sample of 20–21 year olds produced some remarkable results. According to the 20–21 year olds, the number of foreigners in their country represents the second major problem in their society. Furthermore, some 30 per cent of those interviewed thought migrant workers to be a threat to the employment of Belgians and more than half (51.9 per cent) did not believe that foreigners would ever adapt to Belgian culture. Yet, overall, the majority of respondents (53.4 per cent) did not have a negative attitude towards immigrants. These results are further complemented by the finding that 25.4 per cent of the 20–21 year olds had negative attitudes towards migrants. Within this group two categories were distinguished: 9 per cent who were "extremely negative" and 16.4 per cent who were "just negative". A more detailed analysis shows that in Flanders some 10 to 15 per cent of this population has racist or fascist attitudes towards foreigners. Finally, this research confirms earlier research of Billiet which put forward the anomie hypothesis. Racist and ethnocentric attitudes result from a condition of anomie, which means that the people involved are poorly integrated in primary social networks of relatives, friends and other close social networks.

As mentioned earlier, the various signs of a growing intolerance towards foreigners in Belgium in general, and Flanders in particular, triggered a wide variety of counter reactions on different levels of policy-making and social action. At the beginning of 1989, shortly after the alarming results of the 1988 elections, the Belgian government appointed a Royal Commissioner for Migrant Affairs. Together with her associates, the Commissioner, Mrs D'hondt, started an intensive campaign, which deepened the national political debate. Several reports which have since been published have received fairly positive reviews in various academic, political and other circles. However, racist groups have felt strongly offended by the Commissioner's actions, and have proclaimed her as the main enemy of their movement. Inevitably, the debate polarized, yet the initiatives of the Commissioner, together with the growing support for extreme right movements, made clear that the issue could no longer be neglected. The Cabinet of the Commissioner formulated a wide variety of economic, political and cultural policy proposals, and Belgian politicians now have a sound base for their decision making and legislative activities. It has taken a long time for the political world to take a stand on racism, but under the influence of the Commissioner's campaign it appears to have been established.

The galvanizing of politicians into action is also the result of the activities of various social movements. During the second half of the 1980s, the peace movement gradually shifted its focus from the famous cruise missile debate towards a discussion on democracy and tolerance. Traditionally, these social movements have strong roots in various kinds of youth organizations and this is the case today. Youth movements constitute a critical environment with respect to the major issues of the day.

One of the central notions which the Cabinet of the Royal Commissioner put forward with respect to the debate concerning the integration of migrants is that of "insertion". This notion was accepted by the Belgian parliament as a point of departure for its future policy vis-à-vis the migrant population. "Insertion" has been described as assimilation with regard to legislation and regulations in respect of the social basic principles that underpin the culture of the host country. These principles are inspired by concepts and practices of "modernity", "emancipation" and "full fledged pluralism" that are characteristic for modern Western states, unambiguous respect for cultural diversity as a basis for mutual enrichment, with reference to all other realms, and the stimulation of active participation of minorities in policy-making activities and goals.

Youth work: a powerful resource in the Flemish community

Youth work in Flanders is a meaningful and powerful resource for the social integration of children, youth and adolescents, from ages of 4 to 25 years. An analysis of the role and function of the variety of youth organizations in the Flemish part of the Belgian community provides the following results:

- the target groups are children, young people and adolescents;
- special efforts are undertaken for youth organizations to be embedded in the "real world";
- youth work always has a "local" relevance: in other words, its relevance is related to the micro-climate of the target group;
- activities are group-orientated: the group atmosphere is of exceptional importance to the activities of youth work;
- all activities have a non-profit character;
- all activities are clearly located in the educational realm and relate to leisure activities; youth work is disconnected from family and school activities and other obligatory environments;
- leaders or facilitators of youth work initiatives are usually relatively young: this means that activity is predominantly run by adolescents or young adults although, in certain service-orientated sectors, young professionals play an important role;
- the number of volunteers in the youth sector is exceptionally high, especially at local and intermediate levels: professionalization at the local level is restricted to some specific fields;
- youth work is a valuable sector with a specific identity: it has its own vision, pedagogy, methods, atmosphere, etc.

In spite of the great variety of initiatives and organizations, common basic elements can be described in the following way.

Youth work aims at authentic expression and emancipation; the process is more important than the product (the educational outcomes) and hence the pedagogy is fairly diffuse in contrast to the principles of school education. Youth work is characterized by a critical attitude towards the dominant value systems at the local level and there is a lack of homogeneity in commitment *vis-à-vis* broader social issues at the macro-level. Youth work always combines a multiplicity of functions such as recreation, animation, education, training, counselling, etc. and as such youth work is quite different from mono-functional provision such as arts academics or sports leagues.

In the course of its historical development, youth work in Flanders has developed a wide variety of sectors and subsectors. The following is an illustration of the main sectors, which have been recognized officially by the Flemish Community (Redig 1993).

(a) Movements for adolescents and young adults

These initiatives came into existence at the end of the nineteenth century when youth as a special category gained social recognition. They had a fairly romantic character until the second half of the twentieth century and lost much of their attraction during the 1990s.

(b) Youth movements

Youth movements came into existence before the Second World War and were strongly value-orientated, attracting a large number of young people. Although appearing outdated, they currently seem to be well supported and against all expectations their membership is growing again. To a certain extent, youth movements function as counter-movements in a consumer society.

(c) Youth clubs

These initiatives are the consequence of the need young people have for a meeting place of their own and activities about which they can autonomously decide.

(d) Creativity workshops

These came into existence as a reaction against the extreme cognitivist one-sidedness of the traditional school system. They emphasize expression via music, dance, drama, painting, etc.

(e) The playground movement

Originally these initiatives functioned as a social correction to unhealthy and unhygienic living conditions in urban areas. Since then they have evolved towards a provision that stimulate free play and advocates the importance of good playground arrangements and environments.

(f) Grab bag activities

Local exploratory events for children and youth organized by the local youth councils and youth service centres.

(g) Youth arts groups

Drama and music groups that operate on a non-professional basis, like children's choirs, youth bands, etc.

(h) Political organizations for adolescents and young adults

A surprising number of youth organizations are affiliated to the existing political parties and develop activities on a local basis.

(i) Youth workers' education

Originally aimed at organizing general education for young people who left school at the age of 14 or 16 years, this has gradually shifted its focus towards the young unemployed or to part-timers on vocational training schemes.

(j) Provision for underprivileged youth

During the 1990s youth work has paid growing attention to specific target groups such as migrant youth, materially poor Belgian children and young people, homosexuals, etc. It is agreed that these target groups require specific methods and a professionalized approach.

Table 6.5 Estimation of membership of and participation in youth work movements and activities.

	Children	Youth	Leaders	Prof. staff	Total*
Youth movements (adolescents)	140,000	40,000	30,000		210,000
Youth movements (young adults)	20,000	2,000			22,000
Youth clubs		60,000	5,000	200	65,000
Creativity workshops	5,700		600		6,300
Music academies	3,900		400		4,300
Playground events	75,000		7,500	50	82,500
Grab bag events	30,000	15,000	450	30	45,450
Youth arts groups	3,000	1,000	360		4,360
Education for young workers				80	
Underprivileged youth	3,000	3,000		370	6,000

*Without professional staff

In spite of the fact that these categories are not exhaustive, Table 6.5 reflects something of the multiplicity of youth work organizations in Flanders. Contrary to some developments in The Netherlands, where the variety was reduced and professionalized, partly within the context of youth club and community work, diversity has remained an important principle in Flanders. Today, the average child or young person, and their parents, have the opportunity to choose from a multiplicity of activities with reference to age groups, methods, ideology, geographical area, youth cultures, time schedules, etc. The multiplicity of small groups encourages the voluntary commitment of young people, young adults, parents and other responsible persons.

With reference to the debate on multi-culturalism and anti-racism, it is important to delineate the current social relevance of youth work. It is possible to consider youth work in Flanders as a "producer" of:

- themes which gradually find their way to broader contexts and sometimes become real social and political issues: youth work is a laboratory of youth cultures and provides a critical analysis of existing norms and values;
- social and political decision-makers: in an analysis of the curriculum vitae of many leading politicians or leaders of old and new social movements (trade unions, the peace movement, the women's movement, environmentalists, etc.) it is possible to note that many of them have roots in youth work organizations; these organizations provided them with their first opportunity to participate in public forums;
- responsible cadres in private sectors: various industries believe youth work involvement is a reliable predicator for professional zeal and responsibility;
- new strategies and methods of education, guidance and counselling: youth work has always been a laboratory for original and flexible methods and techniques; schools and social workers have often eagerly imported innovations from the youth work sector.

Youth work for multi-culturalism and anti-racism

The above description of youth work in Flanders shows that it is a potentially powerful force in the struggle against racism and intolerance. Yet one should not be too naive. Youth work in Flanders represents in its own organizations, various tendencies and ideologies. This means that racism and intolerance among young people is part of the everyday experience of some youth work organizations, like youth clubs and movements. Recent research by Bral (1991) examining the opinions and attitudes of young people aged 15 years and over, and members of Christian youth movements in Flanders, gives some indication that within these movements racist opinions are alive, just as they are in society at large. This means that those who try to use youth work as an instrument of anti-racist and multicultural education will, to a certain extent, be counteracted by people who have opposing views.

However, these observations should not lead to pessimism. The above-mentioned sociological research findings show that people who are integrated in lively social networks tend to demonstrate more respect towards foreigners than people who live in conditions of anomie. Hence, the existence of networks in youth organizations are an important factor in contributing to the establishment of a tolerant society. Additionally, some special efforts can be made to give these social processes an extra dimension. In this respect, we agree with the Royal Commissioner's invitation to youth work to elaborate actions in a threefold way (Anon 1992). First, youth organizations should foster sensitivity for foreign cultures. Therefore, it is necessary that "intercultural education" becomes an integral and explicit aspect of youth work activities. Hence, the creative elaboration of methods and techniques of intercultural learning is one of the major challenges to youth work volunteers and professionals. Second, the Commissioner suggests building bridges between those youth work organizations that until now were fairly self-indulgent. In particular, regular contacts between indigenous and migrant youth

140

work organizations are necessary. At the local level, the local youth councils, youth services and regional integration centres could play a major role in organizing these processes. This challenge opens opportunities for youth councils at the community level to acquire a qualitatively new dimension. Finally, if youth organizations aim at integrating migrant groups in their activities, they will have to show respect for the different cultural backgrounds of members of this target group. All kinds of barriers such as unfamiliarity with participation costs, mixed activities, overnight stays away from home, etc. will gradually have to be overcome. According to the Commissioner, youth organizations which deliver special efforts in this respect deserve extra financial and professional stimuli.

Elaborating the Commissioner's suggestions further, we can identify four major orientations for anti-racist and multi-cultural youth work:

1. An overall attention to issues of injustice. The majority of youth work organizations have a special sensitivity with respect to problems of injustice, discrimination, etc. In many sub-sectors of youth work, the values of multi-culturalism are supported and defended in a self-evident manner. In the larger movements the annual themes that structure the programmes often refer to these issues. Similarly the participation of youth organizations in various kinds of action, on a local and national level, illustrates their commitment to issues of social justice and solidarity with the materially poor here and in developing countries. Many of these actions would lose much of their strength and significance if youth work organizations did not participate. Through a combination of information, education and action, youth work continues to appeal to feelings and arguments for solidarity. Nevertheless, it is not always easy to realize these ambitions. There is often a tension between the cadres of these organizations and the participants or members at grassroots level. Youth workers need to search continuously for a careful balance between the wider role of the organization and the need for interaction

with young people.

2. Special attention should be paid to economically poor groups. In its activities mainstream youth work in Flanders often tries to work with children and young people who are recognized as being poor. Unfortunately these activities are not always successful. The Royal Commissioner is right to observe that there is still a large gap between the everyday culture of Flemish youth work and the culture of poorer groups. Youth work in Flanders has a strong middle-class character and as such it reflects to a certain extent the values of this dominant group. This does not mean that youth organizations have no chance to cross their own borders or break through their boundaries. Together with sports initiatives, youth work organizations, in principle, offer the best opportunities for spontaneous processes of integration or "insertion", as their activities are mostly informal and leisure-time related. In practice, however, there is still a lot to be done. Gradually, the youth movements in Flanders are paying special attention to the issue. Some have formed autonomous groups for migrants, and as such reflect experiments in self-organization. Others have engaged professionals drawn from the migrant population. Similarly, youth clubs are concerned about the issue because at times they are confronted with racist feelings and activities. Until now professional youth workers have been actively involved in different kinds of training activities. It would be very valuable if the results of these training activities and other forms of exchange of experiences among professionals and volunteers resulted in more systematic analysis, strategies, methods and techniques of anti-racist youth work. In relation to this the work of Deraeck (1992) is valuable.

3. Initiatives that focus on the target group of young migrants could be supported. This type of specialist youth work requires a specific approach. Two such approaches are:
   (a) A natural approach which results mainly from the territorial location of the initiative. For example, a youth movement

or a youth club (re)orientates its activities in a neighbourhood where a high proportion of materially poor families live. In this case the approach comes about in a more or less spontaneous way, sometimes from the very start of the specific initiative, sometimes as a result of changing conditions in a specific area (immigration, social housing projects, etc).

(b) An "instrumental" approach. Here the initiative is an instrument in the struggle against poverty. In these cases new initiatives are created or existing initiatives are reorientated.

The specialized initiatives have developed a characteristic profile over the years, sharing the basic characteristics of the majority of youth work organizations: group work; leisure related activities; a value-orientated character; a combination of functions; participatory decision-making, etc. In spite of the predominant leisure-time orientation, the activities of these specialized initiatives have a much wider scope than is the case in traditional organizations. This is the result of an integrative approach, with guidance and counselling activities with reference to school and/or work, prevention work, outreach work, and health and welfare support, all playing a role. The specific character of these initiatives is also due to a rapid professionalization of this sector of youth work. Specialization implies professionalization, especially in relation to the target group. However, this specialization could also result in a new type of segregation in the youth work sector. Since the early 1990s there has been a definite move towards both general and specific youth work. These tendencies should be carefully analysed and discussed. Perhaps the question needs asking as to whether there is, or should be, a formal distinction between specific and general youth work. Does this enhance segregation or is this a necessary step towards the self-organization of specific groups?

4. This debate makes clear that one can locate intercultural youth work activities on a continuum representing a variety of possibilities. At the one end of the continuum there is a form of youth work which only implicitly involves integrative

activities. At the other end it is possible to find the highly specialized and professional initiatives focusing on specific target groups. Everyday youth work in Flanders is located between these extremes. The geographical location, the tradition or the subsector to which an initiative belongs determines the extent to which materially poor young individuals and groups are reached. Youth movements in urban areas are increasingly reaching such young people living in these communities. Similarly, the playground movement has from its inception paid particular attention to materially poor young people.

Conclusion

This chapter has drawn a picture of youth work in Flanders and outlined how we think this can contribute to containing the increase of racist activity in the region. Policy and practice has emphasized the instrumental nature of youth work to solve various social problems. Yet youth work has a responsibility towards society and has always played an important role in social integration. Our examination has identified racism as a consequence of isolation of specific groups in our society. Flemish society, just like other "advanced" societies in Europe, tends to become a dual society producing conditions of underprivilege. Racism, as a tendency, correlates strongly with conditions of anomie. Hence, the problem of racism should, in the first instance, be solved by overcoming these dualist tendencies. At the same time, in the sociocultural domain, youth work represents a vast reservoir of integrative networks and activities. The strengthening of these networks and activities has a value of its own and can be important in the struggle against racism. Finally, specialized efforts will have to be made with respect to specific target groups. It is not clear yet to what extent these general and specific efforts should be separated or integrated at the level of youth work policy making. The debate on this is continuing.

References and further reading

Anon 1989. *Integratiebeleid: een werk van lange adem*. Rapport van het Koninklijk Commissariaat voor het Migrantenbeleid, deel 1: *Bakens en eerste voorstellen*, deel 2: *Feiten en toelichting van de voorstellen*. Brussels.

Anon 1992. Oog voor de jeugd met visie op morgen: voor een jeugdbeleid dat integraal rekening houdt met de jongeren van andersetnische afkomst. Brussels: Koninklijk Commissariaat voor het Migrantenbeleid.

Billiet, J., A. Carton & R. Huys 1990. *Onbekend of onbemind. Een sociologisch onderzoek naar de houding van de Belgen tegenover de migranten*. Katholieke Universiteit Leuven: Departement Sociologie (SOI)

Bral, L. 1991. *Jeugd in beweging. Een jeugdbewegingsonderzoek bij groepen, leiding en 15-jarigen*. Brussels: Kathlieke Jeugdraad.

Deraeck, G. 1992. *In-kleuren. Perspectieven voor interculturele communicatie*. Leuven: Acco.

Redig, G. 1993. *Jeugdwerk. Het machtig reservoir*. Aartselaar: VVJ.

Waege, H. 1991. *Jongeren en migranten: persmededeling*. Katholieke Universiteit Leuven: Departement Sociologie.

Index